S P E C I A L P R A I S E F O R

Leave the Light On

"There are few books about lesbians in recovery. This is, by far, the best I've read. Those of us who work in the narrow niche of LGBT recovery know the connection between the twelve-step recovery process and the process of "coming out." Jennifer skillfully blends the two together in this memoir. Every gay and lesbian person in early recovery needs to read this book to know they are not alone in their experience. What a gift to our community!

Joe Amico
President, National Association of Lesbian
and Gay Addiction Professionals (NALGAP)

★ ★ ★

"By generously sharing her story in *Leave the Light On,* Jennifer Storm adds to the literature of recovery and hope so helpful for those who think they are alone in their journey. This memoir is a welcome addition to anyone's recovery bookshelf."

Kate Clinton
Comedian and author of *I Told You So,
Don't Get Me Started,* and *What the L?*

★ ★ ★

"The odds of substance use for lesbian, gay, bisexual, and transgender youth are on average 190 percent higher than for heterosexual youth, according to a study by the University of Pittsburgh. Jennifer's touching memoir of addiction and recovery is something that resonated with my life, and I'm sure for many others as well."

Charles Robbins
CEO, The Trevor Project, a non-profit organization
focused on crisis and suicide prevention efforts among lesbian,
gay, bisexual, transgender, and questioning youth

★ ★ ★

"For someone who found recovery fairly late in life (I was 42), I find Ms. Storm's struggles over her addiction at such an early age especially courageous. Peer pressure to "keep the party going" is so strong at her age. She is a shining example of the power of recovery for youth. I applaud her and hope this book brings the treasures of a life in recovery to many, many young people."

Leslie Jordan
Emmy Award-winning actor
and author of *My Trip Down the Pink Carpet*

★ ★ ★

"Jennifer takes the recovery world "by storm" in this gripping account of her struggle with self-destruction and self-acceptance. In *Leave the Light On*, Ms. Storm offers her readers an accessible, honest, and intimate account of the unique challenges faced by those whose recovery as substance abusers is dependent upon honest exploration and loving resolution of their sexual histories and identities. By sharing her own story, Jennifer lays the groundwork for others to follow. It's a book that every clinician who works in the field of addiction and every person who hopes to find recovery can benefit from reading."

Paul L. Hokemeyer, JD, PhD(c)
Licensed Marriage and Family Therapist
The Caron Treatment Centers

LEAVE THE
LIGHT ON

A MEMOIR OF RECOVERY AND SELF-DISCOVERY

BY JENNIFER STORM

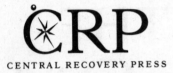

CENTRAL RECOVERY PRESS

CENTRAL RECOVERY PRESS

Central Recovery Press (CRP) is committed to publishing exceptional material addressing addiction treatment, recovery, and behavioral health care, including original and quality books, audio/visual communications, and web-based new media. Through a diverse selection of titles, it seeks to impact the behavioral health care field with a broad range of unique resources for professionals, recovering individuals, and their families. For more information, visit www. centralrecoverypress.com.

Central Recovery Press, Las Vegas, NV 89129
© 2010 by Jennifer Storm

ISBN-13: 978-0-9818482-2-8
ISBN-10: 0-9818482-2-2

16 15 14 13 12 11 10   1 2 3 4 5

Publisher: Central Recovery Press
              3371 N Buffalo Drive
              Las Vegas, NV 89129

Publisher's Note: To protect their anonymity, the names of some of the people in this book have been changed.

Cover design and interior by Sara Streifel, Think Creative Design

In loving memory of Mara Jean Storm

*This book is dedicated to my Higher Power and
the rooms of recovery, for without the combination of these
two powerful entities in my life I would not be here.
To the alcoholic or addict who is still sick and suffering,
may this book read as a hopeful guide to recovery
for whatever you are going through. May you
find hope in these pages.*

To Melissa and Rose, may you both respectively rest in peace.

*To anyone who has ever loved an addict,
I encourage you to never give up and to always
leave the light on in the hope that
it will guide them home.*

CONTENTS

PREFACE

THIS BOOK IS FOR ALL THOSE WHO HAVE READ THE plethora of books out there on addiction and recovery that end with the person entering a rehabilitation program, quitting cold turkey, or simply not stopping the behavior at all—leaving you to wonder, what happened? My first book, *Blackout Girl: Growing Up and Drying Out in America*, published by Hazelden in 2008, was one of those books. I wrote of my addiction to drugs and alcohol, which started at age twelve after I was raped. I proceeded to follow a path of absolute destruction for the ten years that followed that pivotal event. I wrote of my struggles and the trials and tribulations that went along with living on the wrong side of society's norms. I also wrote of my decision to enter a rehabilitation facility and of my first few months in treatment. I flashed back and forth a bit from that time to ten years later, when I was still living a life in recovery that was filled with joy and success beyond my wildest dreams.

But what of the years in between? Where are the books on how one actually *lives* in recovery? They are few and far between, because the rough roller coaster of addiction is much more appealing to our society's thirst for drama than the years of recovery that must come after the ride ends in order for one to truly survive. This book is my survival story as it continued into my first years of attendance in college, my first relationships, and my emotional upheavals as I dealt with my demons—the monsters that lived in my head and that had driven me to drink and to use other drugs in the first place.

After I was raped, I began choosing dark paths. It was as though I was drawn to trouble, addicted to the thrill of defeat rather than the pursuit of anything good or happy. If two paths were placed in a clearing in front of me, but one had danger signs all over as it curved into darkness while the other was straight and clear with a bright light at the end, I would always choose the dark path. My gut would scream, "Go toward the light!" But my feet would veer off onto the curvy, dangerous path that only brought more darkness into my soul and more pain into my life. I never chose the path of least resistance. I fought my entire life, fought unnecessary battles against myself and everyone who crossed my dark path. Those choices kept me living a life in the dark. I was in the dark about my sexuality, my addiction, and my emotional pain caused by sexual assault and the premature losses of people I loved to death and suicide. I hid everything and kept myself numb to all of life's hardships. I welcomed them into my life rather than pushing them away. I invited trouble, thrived on it, and embraced the messes that always followed my careless decisions.

The messes created yet another reason why I should escape and get high or drunk. The cycle of bad choices, initially, was a cycle I placed myself in voluntarily, partly for my own survival. As a young person, I just didn't know how to face the pain in my soul from being raped, so I hid it. I also hid the knowledge that I was gay, and I hid the loathing I had for myself. As I grew more mature and gained the ability to face these demons if I chose to, I was already too deep in the destructive ways I had created to summon up the courage I would have needed to face anything. It was so much easier to just escape—to choose darkness over potential light.

Today I choose the light. Early in my recovery, that wasn't entirely an option; but as lights of knowledge began to flicker in my mind, I knew I could never return to the dark places I had lived in before. As a rape survivor and recovering addict beginning to face my own demons, light became a part of my survival in many ways. For the first years of my recovery, I left the light on at night. I couldn't sleep or feel safe without that light on. Light provided me with a sense of security and well-being, so ultimately I could choose the path with the light at the end of the tunnel. Now I bask in the sunshine of my newfound freedom, joy, and happiness. Darkness is no longer an option for me or a desire, thanks to working a program of recovery.

ACKNOWLEDGMENTS

To my family, as always, for providing me with hours upon hours of support, laughter, unconditional love, and insanity! James and Patricia Storm, Brian Storm, James K. Storm Jr. Love you all!

Cynthia Romano, thank you.

My two beautiful inspirations, Cheyanne and Mia Storm. You are both my sweet angels.

My sponsor, Magi, and her amazing girls, Morgan and Jordan, who kept me sane in early recovery and who continue to serve as daily touchstones for me in my life.

All those who made this book a possibility, Central Recovery Press and Nancy Schenck, Valerie Killeen, Ben Campbell, and Bob Gray for reaching out to me and making this book happen! Jean Cook for your amazing editing skills and constant support and encouragement of my writing, thank you! Sharon Castlen for staying by my side and being an amazing friend and supporter of my work. Devra Ann Jacobs, my agent, for believing in my work and me! Cathy Renna for your mad skills and connections! Jennifer Merchant, you are my ambassador of public relations and my birthday sista. I got mad love for you, girl.

As always, my incredible staff at Victim/Witness Assistance Program and my board of directors; your encouragement, space, and support mean the world to me.

INTRODUCTION

I USED TO LIVE MY LIFE DEEP INSIDE THE VORTEX OF addiction. My life spun and spun out of control for ten years as I plunged further down the scale of disgrace and detriment. I picked up my first drink at age twelve and drank addictively the minute the liquid spilled down my throat. It was as though I had been dehydrated for the first twelve years of my life, and suddenly my mirage appeared in the shape of a tall tin can of beer. I blacked out that first time, and when I woke up I was being sexually assaulted by a man more than twice my age. Thus my introduction to sex and alcohol came in its most destructive and painful manner. Instead of that crime serving as a deterrent from alcohol, it drove me right to the bottle, searching and longing desperately to ease the ache and to quiet the confusion.

I had my first overdose/suicide attempt at age thirteen. What should have been a carefree summer leading to junior high, I wound up spending in a psych ward. Drinking quickly led to smoking pot, dropping acid, and snorting cocaine—which became a weekend norm by age seventeen. I was a bad drunk. I couldn't hold my liquor. "Beer before liquor, never sicker; liquor before beer, you're in the clear"—this age-old saying didn't apply to me. It didn't matter in what controlled combination I attempted to drink; two things were certain: I had no control, and I was always sick as a dog, puking my brains out. That is, until I found cocaine. Cocaine became my great love. It became my savior. It became the great enabler I was looking for. It allowed me to drink more, longer, and stronger. I became dependent upon the combination of drinking and cocaine. It was always about the alcohol, and cocaine gave me the freedom to drink as much as I wanted. I was looking for anything that helped me dull the pain and escape the disorder in my life. I went to great lengths to maintain a chemically induced state of euphoria.

Drinking that way led me straight into more victimization. One day, after discovering for the seventh time in three years that another person I loved was dead, I tried the drug that brought me directly to my knees. I was addicted to crack cocaine before I exhaled my first hit. It engulfed me in a state of nothingness that I demanded at the time. Daily I hit the pipe. I lost many jobs, friends, relationships. I was totally unstable and my life was completely unmanageable.

I drank to avoid dealing with my feelings. Emotions were a foreign concept to me. I quelled them, squashed them, and attempted to create a fantasy world where all things were happy. Except that it wasn't real. I don't think I ever experienced a real emotion. It's not that I didn't feel—emotions would rise in me like a great tide, building and building, with waves of sadness or anger crashing over me—but I would immediately detach. Go somewhere safe in my mind. Or hit a pipe. Or take a drink. Anything to escape and create a state of flat affect that became synonymous with my day.

I was an escape artist.

But I never got away.

Everywhere I went, I was still there.

My emotions were all stuffed inside me, hidden just beneath the surface, encased in darkness like a box of valentine chocolates. Some were darker than others. All were contained and appeared pretty and normal on the outside, but when people tried to scratch beneath the surface, they would find a sticky mess. It became harder and harder to keep my feelings hidden beneath the protective glaze I gave them with my daily dose of whatever substance was most convenient.

Eventually it became impossible to tame the rising surge of shame, guilt, remorse, horror, self-loathing, denial, defeat, despair, and hell I was living in for the ten years I used and abused. All those avoided emotions came to an abrupt head one night after a weekend bender. They wanted out like caged animals and began seeping through every pore of my being. No matter how much I drank, how many hits I took off the pipe—they wouldn't stop coming out. Tears spilled uncontrollably down my face. Anger reddened my cheeks and ears. I sat with a pretty pink razor with daisies on it, slicing and dicing my own wrists apart. Intent upon ending it all, I turned my mattress into what looked like a blood-soaked maxi pad.

The feelings were released and exposed to light. When I woke up the next day in a hospital bed, I was amazed and changed. I had an awakening. It wasn't a moment of clarity, but undeniably an awakening, for it lasted well over a moment. I began hearing what people said around me. I became willing to listen. Words like "alcoholic" and "drug addict" passed my lips with ease. I just knew I was. I was addicted. I was alive. I had a chance. I had hope.

KEEPING IT SIMPLE

The beauty of recovery

was that it was mine and mine alone.

I charted my path as it suited me.

I

Floating on the Pink Cloud

"Our Father who art in heaven, hallowed be Thy name. Thy kingdom come, Thy will be done, on earth as it is in heaven. Give us… give us…" Blood was dripping over my fingers that were clutched tightly around a rosary—the rosary that had been handed down by generations of emotionally unstable women, the rosary I was trying to use to connect to a God whom I never really spoke to until this moment as I screamed out, "Give us… give us…" Frustration overcame me when I couldn't remember the words. My grip tightened until I couldn't distinguish the blood running out of the gaping wounds in my wrists from the blood emerging from slices the crucifix was making. Suddenly the wound, the gaping space of black emptiness in my left wrist, came alive and began to breathe. I realized in horror that the gap wasn't breathing; it was laughing. It had taken on a lifelike shape. The violent gash I had just created with a pretty pink razor was erupting like a volcano, laughing and spattering blood everywhere. Then it began chanting, "Our Father, Our Father" in a childlike, mocking tone, as if it were taunting me for my inability to complete the prayer—or the deed.

My body bolted upright in bed as I was violently ripped from the nightmare. Sweat beads slowly traveled down my spine as my eyes attempted to adjust to my surroundings. Immediately my right hand found my left wrist, and my fingers gently traced the soft, raised pink scars that had begun to close the flesh I had torn apart only months before in a desperate attempt to take my life. I drew a deep breath into my lungs as I pulled my knees to my chest, hugged my arms around them, and slowly exhaled, thanking God it was only a dream. It was a dream that wakened me all too often, although it was the memory inside the dream that made it worse to deal with. I slowly looked around the room for the clock. I didn't have my glasses, so everything around me was out of focus. I saw a bright red, fuzzy blur of numbers but couldn't make them out. I squinted tightly to try and focus my eyes around the numbers, but it was no use. I found my glasses on the table and placed them on my nose. As the lenses dropped down over my tired eyes, they revealed 6:30 a.m. in a bold, red glow. I was still so used to getting up early from being in a structured living environment for the past eighty-odd days that it *almost* felt normal to be awake at this hour.

Two things hit me simultaneously: I was alive, and I was safe. These two things I must constantly remind myself of, and they still feel slightly surprising, especially when I'm awakening from the nightmares of my past. God, the nightmares had been awful. They are little reruns of the horror show of my addiction, my fear, and my desperation that drove me to the last night I used. These mini-movies danced around in my subconscious, and I would have given anything to cancel the upcoming repeat performance.

I was living in Matthew's home. Matthew was a guy I met in the rehabilitation program I had been in for twenty-eight days. We weren't supposed to be dating because the rules of recovery dictate no intimate relationships or major changes for the first year. I was still breaking rules. That much hadn't changed. I moved in with him and his father in State College, Pennsylvania, after leaving the halfway house in Lancaster and lived in the room that was his sister's until she moved out when she got married. Matthew and I were dating, if that is what you want to label it. I had no idea what we were doing because I had no idea from day to day or moment to moment what I was doing. What I wanted and who I was were total mysteries to me. I was catapulted into this new life and these new surroundings, and I felt as awkward as a newborn fawn trying out its legs for the first time, all wobbly and unsure. At least a fawn has its mother's safe underbelly to retreat to when it is unsure. I was here virtually alone.

I swung my feet over the bed and stumbled out toward the hallway. I heard the clanging of coffee mugs in the kitchen to my right, and I knew Matthew and his father were most likely getting ready for work. They had jobs, purpose, and something structured to look forward to. Me, I was twenty-two years old and still floating around in this bubble, this "pink cloud" they call early recovery. I had yet to find a job or purpose or anything other than my daily twelve-step meetings and *Oprah* to keep me sane.

My days had been pretty boring as I adjusted to living outside the daily grind of confinement. I went from having every hour structured with activities that I had to complete or else, to a freedom that didn't quite fit yet. I felt incredibly vulnerable and naked all the time. Like a snail slowly poking its head out into the world for the first time, I realized the world was way bigger and scarier than the comfort of my shell, and I quickly retreated back. I would normally just crawl back into bed and pull the sheets over my head like the snail; but unlike me, the snail doesn't have a horror flick waiting inside its shell. Best to avoid sleep. At least while I was awake I could stop most of the nightmares or quickly disengage them when they flooded my memory like flash photography, quickly blinding me and shifting my balance.

Anyone who tells you early recovery is easy is full of shit. It is the hardest transition and transformation I have ever made in my life. And it never ends. The processing, the talking, the crying, the feeling never stops or I will stop—stop being clean and in recovery, that is. And for me, that would mean to stop living. I was saved somehow from the desire to use and from the survival instinct to run from everything. Now it was my job to maintain the new life that I had been given and to build upon it—to stop running. I felt like that new life was a direct gift from God, and violating that gift by using would be like giving a big ol' middle finger to my higher power, and I was not willing to do that. Even though I was not sure who my higher power was, I was pretty sure I didn't want to piss off him or her just yet.

Recovery is the biggest commitment I have ever made. It is a lifelong changing of behavior and a full shift in thinking. I had to become willing to set aside all I ever thought I knew and open my mind to new ideas and approaches and a completely different way of thinking. It required a deep level of humility and willingness to accept that my ideas and my thinking weren't the best at times. These are tough things for the ego to deal with and let go of. I was more comfortable being right and being stubborn about how right I was. I liked to argue, and I was creative and quick in my intellectual debates. I could make a case for anything and have it come across sounding accurate. I have the gift of bullshit, like most addicts and attorneys. The beauty and sometimes-annoying reality of recovery is that I am not unique in this gift, and, as the old saying goes, "you can't shit a shitter." I had to be willing to put that aside and try to be open to accept that I was wrong and then listen to someone else tell me what was right. Well, that was just exhausting. But it was a process, and one with a built-in learning curve. I had a "get-out-of-jail-free card" to make mistakes and have someone guide me through those mistakes and show me how to do it differently the next time.

I finally figured out in rehab that my problems and my pain stemmed from using alcohol and drugs. That was a huge admission for me. I never wanted to look at using as the problem—in my mind, it was the solution. But after I tried to kill myself, it became abundantly clear to me that using would eventually kill me. Then, as the clarity kept coming, it became easier for me to look back on my destructive years and realize that the majority of bad things that happened in my life involved drugs and alcohol in some way. My actions were at the root of all the evil. These revelations began to light up in my head all at once, and it hit me: I am an addict. I made that admission rather quickly in rehab. I realized I was powerless over drinking as I sat thinking about how often I was actually able to drink and not get hammered. I think I counted about five times. I remembered them vividly, because every time I had obsessed over wanting to drink more. By the time rehab came to an end, I'd had so many lightbulb moments that I felt like a Lite-Brite toy, walking around with all my knowledge beaming out of me. I was glowing with new information that began to transform itself into actual strength within me. They say knowledge is power. What a truth!

As I became more knowledgeable about my disease—and I do believe addiction is a disease—I was building my strength and flexing my new muscles. See, once I knew and understood my enemy, it would be much easier to defeat it. Now that I knew my weakness was the disease of addiction, I began to build my army to protect myself against it. My army consisted of twelve-step meetings, the recovery text of my twelve-step fellowship, my connection to a higher power and praying, continual education for my brain, talking to people, exposing my disease, and just being honest with myself and others. These little soldiers helped me one day at a time in the big war against my addiction. And the soldiers began winning. They are armed not with my hands, but with thoughts in my head. But like any war and any fight, my resources become depleted quickly, and I often need a ton of support to keep winning.

Tired and in need of that support, I found it in State College, a little town up on a mountain in Pennsylvania. Until that point, my

natural reflex in response to everything challenging in my life was
to run, hide, get high, and just escape. This whole idea of facing
everything was a new learned behavior, and like any learned behavior,
practice would make perfect. But the practice, while exhilarating at
times, was also horrifically draining.

State College is home to Pennsylvania State University and not
much else. The town thrives on the university, and if you live there you
are a student, faculty member, staff, or an unfortunate townie who was
born there and somehow ended up never leaving. I joked that State
College was a fairy-tale land, a little make-believe oasis way up over a
mountain in a valley—"Happy Valley," to quote the town's slogan. The
town had very little crime, at least little that the residents wanted you
to know about, though date rapes and assaults occurred on campus and
were underreported or never reported. The town also had very little,
if any, homelessness or poverty, unless you counted the small trailer
park next to the local Wal-Mart or the one long-haired dude we called
the vagrant who wandered the streets. One lady also wandered the
streets; we called her the dime lady because she walked around picking
up change all over town. The story was that she was very wealthy but
chose to live on the streets because of mental health issues. Otherwise,
students, professionals, and a bunch of drunks and former drug addicts
made up the population of Happy Valley.

There were no drug dealers or prostitutes on the streets at night.
I learned later that they hide in the fraternity houses surrounding the
campus. After all, there are always drugs to be found; you just have to
have the ability to sniff them out like a trained dog. I'd always had that
uncanny ability. No matter where I was, I could sniff out a drug user
a mile away and would find myself migrating in that direction. It's a
gift, really—just one I no longer have any use for, unless you consider
the Drug Enforcement Administration (DEA). I would be a great drug
enforcement agent because my nose for drugs is ten times better than
any trained bloodhound's. Actually, if the DEA agents were smart, they
would recruit at rehabs, because who better to hunt down drug dealers

than their best customers? Perhaps ironically, you cannot be in the DEA, FBI, or CIA if you answer yes to these questions:

Have you done illegal drugs in the past ten years?

(Okay, if I wait this one out, maybe I can enlist.)

Have you smoked marijuana fifteen times or more in your lifetime?

(Ummm, I've smoked that much in a day.)

Application DENIED!

Guess I won't be joining the force anytime soon. Regardless, State College was a quaint, peaceful town. It truly was Happy Valley to me upon my arrival. I was more than four hours away from my former life in Allentown. Walking the streets, I had a freedom that felt incredible to me. Bad memories and potential dangers weren't lurking around every corner. Everything was fresh and new and clean, like a crisp piece of white paper just waiting to be filled with adventures. I would later find out that avoiding downtown on Thursday, Friday, and Saturday nights after about 10:00 p.m. would serve me well, because at those times the streets were filled with drunken students and alumni celebrating the latest football win or drowning their sorrows over the latest loss—reactions that looked oddly the same. Otherwise, it was the perfect place for me to start my life over. It felt safe, for now.

I was flying high on what they call in early recovery the "pink cloud." The pink cloud is a common place for many newcomers to land in the beginning of recovery, because it really is a different type of "high" to discover how wonderful life can be without chemicals. When you accept the realization that you never again have to live the way you were living in that utter darkness, it is amazing! You begin to feel alive again. For the first time, your skin is breathing. Your senses are awakened in a whole new way. Food tastes different, flowers smell pretty, the sky is just a little bit bluer, and the possibilities begin to seem endless. Everything is so new, so bright, so exciting that you feel like a little kid again, and in many ways, most of us are. Learning to walk and talk again in recovery is such an amazing gift. Tears are genuine, and they flow freely like rain. Feelings are actually felt in their fullest states. Music floats differently into the ears and sounds crisper, and lyrics make sense on a deeper level. Laughter is the real, heartfelt, stomach-hurting kind of pure laughter. Life is lived. A day has a definite beginning and end. Morning gives way to evening and all is remembered and experiences are wholly felt. Lips actually enjoy touching the cheek, while smiles splash across the face and are felt deep inside the heart. Blackouts aren't an option; missing pieces of the night before isn't a possibility.

I was loving everyone in the rooms of my twelve-step meetings, loving being alive, and loving my sheer existence. I had the innocence of a newborn and a naiveté that was out of sync with my past "been around the block, don't mess with me" persona. A new lease on life was what I signed in rehab and it felt wonderful, as though I could breathe a huge sigh of relief because my past was miles behind me. My most horrible nightmares and trashy actions were left sitting on top of the mountain where my rehab was located or were hidden in my sleep or in my mind where only I could see them.

So I was free—free to begin a new life, to start over fresh and, I hoped, to not screw up royally.

2

LYRICAL RANTS

KATHY WAS, HANDS-DOWN, MY ABSOLUTE BEST FRIEND throughout my early twenties. We met during high school when I had a job at a local low-end clothing store for teens. She was my manager and was a couple of years older than I was. We both had a love of partying that we recognized in each other during early Saturday morning openings when we would both stumble in hung over as hell. We would glance up at each other and exchange the same glassy-eyed, nauseated expression, which made us fast best friends. We attended rival high schools, so we didn't know many of the same people. It was nice to have a friend outside my inner circle.

Ours was the annoying kind of friendship where if we weren't in each other's immediate company, we were glued to the phone talking endlessly about anything and everything at all hours. The only time we would break from conversation was to shower before meeting up with one another, and I am pretty convinced that if I'd had a phone in the shower, we would have been talking then too. It got so bad that finally my parents got me my own phone line in the house. Kathy also had her own line, so that freed us up to talk incessantly. We talked about everything girls our age talked about: clothing, fashion, boys, friends, relationships, work, dreams, etc. We analyzed everything together and wouldn't have dreamed of leaving the house to meet up without getting verbal acceptance of what we were wearing that night. At that time, she was the closest thing I'd ever had to a sister. We trusted each other with everything in the way only young girls do.

I was never physically attracted to her, as I had been with some of my other best friends. Not because she wasn't a beautiful girl, but because it just wasn't there for me. She was truly my best friend and that was it. We started hanging out every weekend, then eventually that began to bleed into the week, and then we were partying hard-core all the time. Kathy and I could party it up just as hard as any guy we knew. We held our own in any situation and got hammered together to the point of oblivion.

One time we decided to hit an all-day beer-tasting festival, where you buy a twelve-ounce glass and walk from booth to booth trying a variety of ales and microbrew beers. It was like a candy store for an alcoholic. Although beer was my main drink of choice, mainly because of accessibility and cost, I wasn't a huge beer fan, and I had never really ventured beyond the cheap shit we could afford to drink in high school. When we wanted to really be tacky and tie one on, we traded up for a forty-ounce malt liquor, with Crazy Horse or Colt 45 among my favorites. So this was new territory for me, and I was excited! We arrived around 11:00 a.m., about an hour after I had woken up, and we bought our little glasses. I was pissed that they only had twelve-ounce glasses; I mean, who the hell drank from a twelve-ounce glass unless it was to do a shot of something? I never went for anything below sixteen ounces, even when I was drinking wine. Yeah, I was that kind of classy drunk; I drank my white zinfandel from a sixteen-ounce beer stein. I was hot—*not*!

We started hitting booths like kids at Halloween, going from booth to booth and sucking down beer, barely tasting the bitter microbrews we were slurping down. After all, we weren't connoisseurs there to savor the aroma and taste; we were there to get drunk quickly and cheaply. The booths were set up in a circle, with about twenty different breweries present. Intermixed with the breweries were traditional German food vendors serving bratwursts and sausages. That meant for a vegetarian like me there was nothing to eat, which was just as well because I was filling up on beer quickly and the yeast was beginning to bloat my stomach.

In the middle of the food and beer, a makeshift stage featured several bands playing throughout the day. By 1:00 p.m., Kathy and I had hit every booth and were dancing our drunken asses off in the middle of the festival to a cover band belting out "Sweet Caroline." Kathy and I were infamous for getting extremely loaded at clubs, pushing our way to the front of the stage like mad groupies and dancing around like absolute fools. We were bouncing off people all around us, but most of them were just as loaded as we were so they didn't mind. We began our own mini-mosh pit while singing at the top of our lungs: "Sweet Caroline, badda dum, good times never seemed so good. *So good! So good!*" The band ended its set after the song, and Kathy and I collapsed onto the stage with our arms around one another in fits of laughter.

The crowd began to disperse back to the various booths around us. The band's crew was pulling equipment off the stage, and I was shamelessly flirting with a stage crew dude when I heard Kathy's drunken voice boom out of the speaker next to my head. She sang, "Sweet Caroline, badda dum, Kathy is feeling mighty fine, badda dum, and Storm's right behind, badda dum." Kathy had a gift for twisting song lyrics to fit the situation we were in. These lyrical rants always sent me into hysterics, and this time was no different. I was drunk on my ass, lying on the stage, holding my stomach, rolling around, and laughing so hard that tears were streaming out of my eyes. After a verse or two, one of the band crew came up to us and politely removed the microphone from Kathy, who slurred a couple of choice swear words at him before finally giving up and collapsing down next to me.

That was typical of our friendship—we were always hammered and always making asses out of ourselves. We spent countless hours in front of the mirror at home making sure each strand of hair was in place and our makeup was done to perfection, and we were always dressed to the nines; but no matter how hard we tried to keep it together, every night we would end up total messes—drunk and falling around, getting as dirty as kindergartners on a playground at recess. The next day we would call one another and compare beer-induced wounds. Kathy was fond of wearing skirts with stockings and would always wind up with a big blowout in her knee from stumbling to the ground. We would often sit in the car outside nightclubs burning a big bowl before entering the club. When we got out of the car, I would look over and she would be gone. I would hear giggling coming from her side of the car and stumble over only to find her lying on the ground after busting her ass on the way out of the vehicle.

She was a riot, and I loved hanging out with her. She was crazy, and she didn't hold back at all. She loved her booze and loved her pot, which gave us incredible but shaky common ground to stand on. Kathy never did coke and wasn't into that scene at all, so that was where we differed a lot. I never told her about how much coke I did. Even when I was high around her, she never knew because she was always just as fucked up on beer or pot. At the nightclubs we went to, I sneaked off and did lines of coke off the toilet in the bathroom and then rejoined Kathy at the bar just in time to slam back another lemon drop, her favorite shot. She was never the wiser, and after she left the bar to head home at closing time, I left to hang out with a different crowd. While Kathy got up to go to work the next day, I was still out partying and blowing off work.

I tried to maintain my friendship with her after I moved to State College. She came to see me in the hospital before I left for rehab, and

I knew she couldn't put words together to explain how weird she felt as she saw my bandages on my wrists, but she never judged me. She just wished me luck and said, "Do whatever you gotta do to get better, kid."

I would see Kathy on my frequent weekend trips to Allentown, but things were weird because she was still out partying. Although I would meet up with her at the local hangouts, it just didn't quite fit me anymore. I really tried to go to bars and pretend I was having fun with everyone. I would have moments of good conversation or a couple good laughs, but they were always followed by my friends reaching the point of intoxication, and then something in the room would change for me. It was as though with each shot and beer they drank, my friends' souls and spirits would slowly leave their bodies. They would appear strange to me, slurring their speech and saying random things that made no sense, yet they expected that I would laugh or respond. But I just couldn't "get it up" for them to laugh on cue. There was no verbal connection whatsoever. I was left feeling blank and hollowed in their presence.

The worst was when people would stumble up to me and ramble on and on about how proud they were of me for being able to be there and not drink. In their own drunken stupors, they would gush over me about how noble and amazing it was that I wasn't drinking. It always made me feel completely uncomfortable and speechless. I usually just nodded, gave a big smile, and said, "Thanks," while I was screaming inside.

That happens still to this day every time I attempt to masquerade out in the land of drunks, which I have done less and less as the years of recovery have piled up in my life. But when I do, it always strikes me as the most hypocritical of all compliments.

Sometimes I wanted to blend in so badly, to just be what the world defines as "normal," that I did some stupid shit that could have gotten me in serious trouble.

3

No Relationships

I WALKED INTO THE KITCHEN TO THE GLORIOUS SMELL of coffee, which is one of my favorite smells in the world. As I slowly poured the dark energy into my mug, I felt Matthew's hands slip around my waist and my body immediately stiffened. He grabbed me close to his body and nuzzled his face into the nape of my neck. My entire insides recoiled as every fiber of my being rejected his touch. I remained stiff and muttered, "Good morning," as I swiftly slipped out of his grasp and moved around the breakfast bar onto the stool facing him.

I stared blankly down at my coffee. I was so incredibly confused by what I was doing with him. I was trying to fill that infamous void—the one I used to pour drugs and alcohol into—with people, more specifically, with Matthew. It was becoming clear to me that we were both just kind of using each other to avoid dealing with reality in its entirety. That had seemed okay while I was in treatment, because

I had already given up so much and our relationship served as a nice distraction. We barely knew each other; we'd only had glimmers of stolen conversations while in rehab together. I didn't know his middle name, what his childhood was like, who his family was, where he went to school. All I knew was that he was going through a similar situation to mine, and we both craved love and attention as though it were air. It felt good to have someone adore me the way he claimed he did. He really acted as though he loved me, even though he barely knew me.

When Matthew got out of rehab, he went directly home instead of going to a halfway house like I did, so he was used to being back in the world and working. He wrote me these long, impassioned letters while I was in the halfway house; it was like he was a soldier off at war and I was his great love. He would send me photos of himself, which his father would take for him, holding up handwritten signs that read, "I miss you and I love you." At the time, I would clutch them to my chest and feed off the energy of the love he sent me.

But now, looking at him from across the kitchen table, I had no idea what I was doing. I didn't love him; I barely knew him. For that matter, I barely knew or loved myself.

Counselors in rehab and anyone else who has more than a year of solid recovery will tell you to avoid getting into a relationship within the first year of recovery, because it only serves to distract you and in many ways replaces the alcohol and drugs. At the time it didn't make sense to me, because the sensation of someone paying me attention outweighed any new information or personal growth I had experienced in rehab. He was good-looking and kind, and my self-esteem was, as usual, in the toilet and solely reliant upon the attention of others. So dating someone in rehab made sense and was a good idea in my problematic way of thinking.

As the cobwebs slowly began to clear in my brain, the idea of a year's abstinence was starting to make a little sense to me. It is easy to hide behind something else, even when you are not using. It is easy to get lost in a relationship, or the idea of one at least, which keeps the mind in denial of all the reasons why it is not a good idea to be in one. As an addict, I looked for anything and everything outside of myself to fill that void I had inside. Men had always been one of those things I had turned to in order to avoid dealing with myself. But the longer I worked a program of recovery and began to explore my past in therapy sessions and group sessions, the more it was starting to make sense to me that I had never really known love, and in many ways love and sex were just vices I used to escape, like alcohol and drugs.

I was beginning to understand that my views on sex and love were just as skewed as all my other views. I was beginning to understand that anyone who would run to a guy in rehab whom she didn't know just because he told her she was pretty was messed up. I sneaked around at night against the rules in rehab to steal quick kisses with some guy I had just met, all because he paid me attention. And that attention was another drug for me—one that I was just learning could be as destructive as using, if I let it. It was becoming clear to me that I had never had a healthy intimate relationship in my life, and my obsession and feelings for Matt were just emotional baggage that I hadn't yet checked in recovery.

We tried to have sex a couple of times, but sex without being drunk or high was incredibly awkward for me. In fact, sex at all was like a foreign concept. I had no idea what real intimacy was because I had never really had sex without being high, and most of my sexual endeavors just left me feeling dirty, used, and empty. After all, my first sexual experience was a rape—a drunken rape. It was no wonder I was a mess in this area.

This only fueled the extreme confusion I already felt regarding sex and my sexuality. From a very early age, kindergarten in fact, I can tell you whom my first crushes were on—girls. I had always had feelings toward girls and never knew it wasn't okay until people in positions of authority so studiously began pointing it out to me when I would express my innocent crushes. I was teased in school as a young girl for making it known that I had feelings toward another girl. I didn't like the taunting. I didn't want to be labeled a freak or abnormal, so I began to fake it.

I had fleeting moments of intimacy that were blurred by total drunkenness, so I was really lost. To avoid dealing with all the uncomfortable feelings that came along with it, I found myself emotionally detaching during sex. I would lay there while he was inside me, moaning on cue, trying to do and say all the things that I thought should be said during sex: "Oh yeah, come on, baby." But I was as flat as an iron. If he tried to look into my eyes, all he would see was a distant, empty void where I imagined true emotions and intimacy should be. Instead of being present, I was off in my safe place of detachment. I would just mentally float away and create visual places where I was free or safe. Sometimes I would be swimming in the ocean and feeling the sunshine on my face. Other times I would be flying high above the clouds and feeling light as a feather, where no one could hurt me. There I didn't have to deal with the fact that someone was invading me and that I didn't enjoy it the way I was told I was supposed to.

Instead, I floated while Matt fucked, as I had always done during sex.

I learned later in therapy that this is a common phenomenon for women who have been sexually assaulted. With my introduction to sex coming in the form of an assault, everything afterward was a mess. How can anyone really expect a person not to be confused? Love and sex got all intermingled and twisted in my head and intrinsically became one for me. I thought sex was supposed to be this uncomfortable obligation I had to offer up to men to gain acceptance and love. I was extremely promiscuous growing up—not because I liked sex, or guys for that matter, but because I thought that was how one obtained love and acceptance. That was what I knew. That was what I had learned. No one taught me differently.

This is where many people get confused about young girls and their behaviors. Often folks just shake their judgmental heads briskly back and forth in disgust at the displays of many misguided young females. What people don't understand or realize is that the majority of the times you see a young girl acting in the manners I did—dressing provocatively, flirting like crazy with any boy that moves—these are clear warning signs or indicators that she was probably at some point sexually abused. She isn't a slut or a whore or another label society would immediately assign out of assumption. She is most likely scared, confused, hurting, and deeply, deeply violated in some way, and she is acting out in the only way she knows how. Young people do not usually verbalize their feelings. I never had the ability to articulate my feelings, but boy, if people had just paid close enough attention to my actions long enough, they would have seen I was really screaming out for help.

I was so screwed up in my head that I used sex as a way to gain attention. The terrible thing was that I never wanted to actually engage in sexual activity. I just wanted someone to pay attention to me, to hold me, to tell me I was pretty and worthy, even to just *see* me. Sex came as part of this deal with most men, because, let's face it, if they think they can get it, they will try. Sex was uncomfortable for me, and most times I hated every second of it, but during those moments at least I wasn't alone. Someone was paying attention to me, and in my mind, I guess, loving me. My idea of love was royally screwed up also. The love I got from my parents had been dysfunctional. My mother would say she loved me while telling me what a bad person I was. And my father, well, he always told me he loved me, but he was rarely around when I needed him.

The love I sought from men was unhealthy and was not love at all, but abuse, lust, sex, and pain. I wouldn't have known what true, unconditional love was if it had come up and slapped me in the face, so how exactly was I supposed to love Matthew? How was I supposed to give him something I didn't possess myself? How was I supposed to love him unconditionally when all the love I had ever received or given was filled with expectations and conditions, whether they were spelled out or in my head?

I didn't know how to tell him I just wanted to be his friend. I couldn't find the words to tell him that, while this was a nice distraction for a while, I was just not into it. I was barely in touch with my own feelings, so how was I to try and explain to him what they were? I never had the ability to communicate my true feelings to people, especially if they were going to be potentially hurt or would hold me accountable in some way. I was incredibly codependent in this way. I would set my feelings or my needs aside, always for the sake of another. I did this even when I wasn't getting anything positive out of a relationship. I didn't know how to break this cycle just yet.

But I knew enough to recognize that this relationship with Matt was potentially as damaging as my substance abuse. I just wasn't quite sure yet how to open my mouth up and allow truth to flow out of it without fearing the outcomes, the rejection, the pain, the guilt. I still wasn't sure how to put myself and my needs first. So I just sipped my coffee as he swooped down and gave me a quick peck on the cheek before he and his father went off to work. I stiffened, and he left the house with no clue that I was sickened to my core.

Whenever he would try to talk to me about "us," I would just smile and say everything was okay. Matt and I would often go to meetings together, and I could tell from the vibe we got from many people in the rooms that our relationship wasn't looked upon fondly. After all, we were each supposed to be focused on ourselves, but it was apparent that we were only focusing on each other.

My father and stepmother weren't thrilled that I was living with a guy at that time either, but they managed to be okay with it because I was sleeping in a separate room. I think in many ways they were just so happy I was not home while trying to learn to maintain my recovery. We all knew my chances for recovery would have been slim at home. They encouraged me every day to find an apartment or place of my own. I needed to do the next right thing and take care of myself. It was becoming clearer that I was going to have to step up to the plate and take a swing—one that would unfortunately hit right in Matt's heart.

4

BAD COFFEE AND HARD CHAIRS

NAVIGATING THIS NEW STATE OF RECOVERY WAS SCARY and I wasn't sure what I wanted to do with my life, so I hung on tightly to a famous slogan in twelve-step fellowships: "Take it one day at a time." Twelve-step slogans are the best because they just bring things home in a simple way, like "Keep it simple, stupid," or "Progress, not perfection." Some of them saved my life and sanity in the first couple of years I was in recovery.

I didn't have a job at first; I thought it would be best to just take it easy for a while. Everything was so strange for me. The world around me felt very large, so I kept my reality based in the rooms of recovery. I worked the Twelve Steps daily by writing, going to meetings, praying at night, and doing a daily inventory of my actions. Each night I would sit down and assess my day and ask myself certain questions: Did I harm anyone today? Was I honest in my encounters with others? Was

I true to myself? Were there any verbal amends I needed to make to anyone? This assessment was a great tool we used in rehab to help keep ourselves accountable in our recovery. After all, I am human and this was a whole new way of life, so making mistakes was common, but it was what I did with those errors in judgment that mattered. Did I learn from the mistake? Did I try to make things right? These were the thoughts that flooded my mind at night before I said my prayers and went to sleep. It certainly made hitting the pillow and drifting off to sleep much easier to do.

I made sure I hit a meeting every day. It was my only connection to people, because usually I stayed in the house watching *Oprah*, smoking cigarettes, and eating everything I could get my hands on. Matt's father was very much a meat-and-potatoes kind of guy, and we lived in a rural area that was not conducive to my vegetarian lifestyle. So I found myself eating junk food—chips, cookies, macaroni and cheese from the box—all food with little nutritional value. Mostly I was eating out of boredom and loneliness.

The meetings I attended were a great way for me to process all the change I was experiencing, and I began to meet new people. There are different types of twelve-step meetings, such as discussion meetings, in which everyone just openly shares; reading meetings, in which the focus is on a passage in a recovery-related book; and speaker meetings, in which a person with more than one year in recovery openly shares about his or her past and how things are now. My first meeting in State College was a Sunday discussion group that met at 3:00 p.m. at St. Andrew's Episcopal Church. Most of the meetings I ended up attending were held there. St. Andrew's was set in the heart of downtown. It was a nice change from the rural area where I was living.

The church was located across the street from a large football field that belonged to the local high school. I would pull up out back and park to find several of my fellow addicts milling about and smoking and chatting. I always came to the meetings early to help set up, make coffee, and arrange recovery literature on the tables. It gave me more to do and an opportunity to meet with others before the meetings. It is suggested in recovery to always arrive fifteen minutes prior to a meeting and stay fifteen minutes afterward to meet-and-greet others. That time is often referred to as the "meeting before and after the meeting," time set aside to get to know one another and discuss not so much our recovery or addiction, but the more personal details of our lives.

I had been to meetings in Lancaster, Allentown, and York, and the great thing I learned about recovery meetings is that no matter where you go, you can walk into any meeting and immediately feel at home. Walking into a meeting, there is a familiarity that I can't really explain. It is like walking into your house after being gone a long time; the furniture may have been moved around a little bit, but the smell and feel remain the same.

The meeting rooms are always set up in a similar manner. Chairs are arranged in a circle, or in rows for a more traditional speaker format. There is always a table covered with twelve-step literature and portions of the fellowship's recovery text that are printed out to be read during the meeting. Posters that display the Twelve Steps and the Twelve Traditions are often hanging on the wall. A daily reflection book, open to that particular day, is often set out for people to read. The aroma of strong coffee is always in the air, and lingering drunks and addicts clinging to their one socially acceptable vice are smoking outside the building. The best way to detect a recovery meeting is by the loitering of smokers outside any church building—they aren't there for Sunday school!

For meetings at St. Andrew's, I entered a huge, auditorium-like room in the church basement that was clearly usually used for larger church functions, such as dinners, because there were tables against the wall and a nice, big kitchen at the end of the room. The familiar large metal coffee urn was always churning out what was probably the worst coffee in history. Caffeine becomes a new addiction after rehab. I became hooked on Mountain Dew, a soda I had never drunk except in the summer when I would blend it with gin, pineapple juice, pineapple chunks, and ice. Hmm, that was quite the refreshing summer beverage. I was a master with a blender in my addiction, always the life of the party making crazy concoctions.

But now I was like my peers, walking into meetings clutching coffee or some other heavily caffeinated beverage. I wasn't alone. Most newcomers (the term for people in early recovery) were also in a caffeine-induced haze. You could always pick us out by our large bottles of soda and the glazed look in our eyes. I took a seat in the circle of metal chairs. Another thing about recovery meetings—not only the worst coffee in the world, but also the most uncomfortable chairs your ass will ever grace, and you're held hostage in them for at least a solid hour. It's a small price to pay, though, considering the surfaces my ass used to fall on during drunken stupors. I was never a graceful drunk, and often found myself at the bottom of a hill or scraping my knee against the pavement of a parking lot after taking a nasty tumble. Or I would be in the filthiest homes, buying and doing drugs in some of the worst neighborhoods. Couches and chairs that held who-knows-what inside would hold me for hours upon hours while I did drugs.

So a metal chair was nothing for me to bear for one small hour.

5

CHECKS AND BALANCES

BEFORE LEAVING THE HALFWAY HOUSE, I WAS TOLD
I must do a ninety-in-ninety, which is to go to ninety meetings in
ninety days, and also immediately get a sponsor to call every night. A
sponsor would walk me through the program of recovery. She would be
my tour guide, she would call me on my shit, and she would try to be a
source of wisdom and comfort to me without being enabling. It's a tall
order, and one that needs to be filled with caution. As usual, being the
"quick to jump to a decision without thinking" kind of gal, I filled that
order with the same reckless abandon I had used to fill my beer glass—
quick and sloppy.

As instructed, I got a sponsor at the first meeting I attended. I was
a good student and wanted to follow my instructions perfectly. You
see, I was also a people pleaser. I wanted to do everything right, which
is impossible. Perfection, while a nice concept, is bullshit. There really

isn't anything *perfect* in this world, although the majority of us are still aiming at, trying for, and seeking it every minute of every day.

So I set out on my quest to find the perfect, Buddha-like sponsor who would usher me flawlessly into this recovery thing. In my first meeting, a woman named Tina spoke and her words struck me. She was in her late thirties with badly bleached, dirty blonde, frizzy hair and a horrible complexion. Her face seemed to be covered in acne scars, which I later learned actually came from her picking her face for hours in the mirror while sketching out in a heroin- and cocaine-induced haze.

I was immediately taken by her as she spoke of her own battle as a cokehead and alcoholic. She smoked a lot of crack, shot heroin, and got into a lot of trouble with the law. She seemed perfect for me! After the meeting, I walked up to her and asked her to be my sponsor and she said yes. To have a sponsor who had also done the drugs I had done and more was so exciting to me. Finally, someone who could relate to me!

I spoke to Tina daily and sought her guidance on everything I did. In rehab, I had learned painfully that my own thinking had gotten me addicted, so it was time to start taking suggestions. One key example they gave me in rehab group therapy was my faulty thinking and my behavior with Matt—my sneaking around and trying to hook up with a guy I knew nothing about. In my head, I thought nothing of what I was doing. Seeing Matt was a convenient distraction for me and something I felt justified in doing because I didn't see the harm in it to myself or others. My counselors and peers in the group abruptly pointed out to me that I was engaging in what they call in recovery "stinking thinking." This is any form of thinking that takes you away from your purpose—the purpose being to maintain recovery. It would take me a long time to start putting these pieces of new information into practice in my life. It was critical for me to have someone with more recovery experience in my life to constantly reinforce these principles in my malfunctioning brain. As with any behavioral change, recovery must be reinforced and practiced daily. In many ways that is what a sponsor is—a behavioral modifier.

The day Tina agreed to be my sponsor, I left the meeting and hopped into my little silver Toyota, one of my possessions that I still managed to have. Although it was falling apart at the seams, it got me from points A to B, which was good because Matthew lived in bumfuck turn left at Egypt, on the outskirts of State College. It took me twenty to thirty minutes to get into town for my meetings. Often I would go to a meeting that was in Center Hall, closer to our house. It was a great little meeting with people who were more rural than the professional types I encountered in State College. In State College everyone held degrees, and those in my meetings were often well-educated and established. They were lawyers, doctors, professors, or other professionals affiliated with the university. In Center Hall, I was among my own type of people—everyday workers with little educational background.

Although the recovery text, meetings, and my sponsor were great for keeping me on track in recovery, I needed more. Like most people with addiction, there were core emotional reasons I was addicted, the majority of which stemmed from my early confusion about my sexuality and my first sexual experience being an assault. Instead of addressing these things, I learned to escape and to hide everything in alcohol and drugs. And though recovery allowed me to look at these reasons and begin to heal, more in-depth counseling was necessary for me to really unearth the entire trauma I had experienced.

Often it is crucial to seek various types of treatment or medications to sustain recovery, and whatever is determined to be the best course of action is the best course of action, period. People in recovery sometimes offer a lot of judgment and misperceptions, including negative reactions toward medications, counseling, and people with a dual diagnosis. There are some who believe twelve-step recovery is the answer and the only answer, but I believe there are others who need more. I have watched people try to go off their meds because of others' disdain for meds in the rooms of recovery, and all it did was drive them back to drink or to engage in other unhealthy behaviors. If people need medications or other treatments to sustain certain chemicals in their brains to obtain and maintain recovery, in my opinion they should listen to their doctors' recommendations. Later on, they can always look for alternatives when they have some time in recovery under their belts.

My take on this was that it was up to me determine what worked for me, in consultation with a sponsor, therapist, doctor, or all three. The beauty of recovery was that it was mine and mine alone. I charted my path as it suited me. There were many road maps placed before me in the rooms of recovery, and many of them worked, so I was beginning to use what applied and let go of what didn't apply for me.

Still on the pink cloud "high" of early recovery, I was ready to learn everything I could and beginning to feel things I had never felt or had refused to feel in the past. Counseling, I thought, would be a great way to help me process my emotions appropriately. In addition to my program of recovery, I needed counseling to dive deep into my past assaults, to take a closer look at my dysfunctional relationship with my mother and how that played into my own addiction, and to really understand *why* I drank and drugged.

I began to see a therapist who was located near St. Andrew's church and was recommended to me by several others in the program. She was a middle-aged woman with whom I felt comfortable almost immediately. She had a wonderful way about her, wasn't judgmental in any way, and put me at ease quickly. We began working together, twice a week at first. I had nothing but time on my hands, and my medical assistance was paying for my therapy, so I was taking advantage of it. We had to establish a time line, and I had to bring her up to speed on my life. That alone was exhausting. It is sometimes so much easier to talk with someone who knows you, but at that time, those people were few and far between in my life. So with every new encounter, I found myself telling my life story again. In hindsight, that was really a good thing because it made me talk about my past and expose my disease constantly and on many different levels. With my therapist this was on the most intimate of levels because she needed to know it all—the good, the bad, and the ugly—to fully understand how my mind worked and how she could begin to help me heal. She continually gave me homework assignments to do so I could see myself more clearly. We talked about everything. I found myself opening up to her easily, and before I knew it the hour was up and it was time for me to leave. She was helping me identify my patterns and understand my personality, both my assets and my flaws.

Between my therapist and my sponsor, I was beginning to have some nice checks and balances in my life that had never been there before. I had people I could confide in and go to for guidance.

6

FINISHING SOMETHING

BECAUSE I DIDN'T HAVE MUCH GOING ON DURING THE
time between my meetings and my therapy sessions, I became obsessed
with Oprah Winfrey. I had always loved her show, and it was one thing
that had bonded my father and me in the past. For whatever reason,
he always made sure he was home by 4:00 p.m. when I got home
from school, and we would watch *Oprah* together. It was nice to have
something that bonded my father and me, because we didn't have a
whole lot in common as I was growing up. I think I just confused and
scared the shit out of him most of the time. He wasn't equipped to deal
with a teenage girl on his own. Since he and my mother divorced after
my sexual assault and he stayed to raise me and my two older brothers,
he was a little lost in the parenting department. He was used to the role
of provider; but with my mother gone, he had to attempt to provide
the more motherly, emotional type of support too. He had no clue how

to do that, so instead we would sit and watch *Oprah* and try to connect through the topics on the show.

It wasn't as though I missed the motherly stuff, because my mother was not your stereotypical mom. She had been verbally abusive and emotionally absent all my life, so to have her physically absent as well didn't seem like that much of a difference to me. When I would act out, as I had become accustomed to doing, my father would tiptoe around me as though I might scream or shatter at any time. In many ways, that was pretty accurate. Back then I was a walking live wire at all times, so no one could ever predict my emotional outbursts or severe mood swings.

So now here I was years later, glued to the TV at 4:00 p.m. each day like an obsessed evangelist watching *The 700 Club*, waiting for my daily dose of scripture. In early recovery, people are like sponges; we soak up everything around us. I would go to my daily meeting and share my newfound Oprah enlightenment, which would always rouse a chuckle out of everyone. In fact, it earned me the nickname "Oprah Jen" for my first year at meetings in Center Hall.

Instead of laughing at me, though, those people understood what I was saying and going through. They understood how new to all this I was and how, in early recovery, everything is a deep and new revelation.

I was starting to go stir-crazy being in the house and not working, so I went to the local hobby store and looked around. Being alone for eight hours or more was too much for me, and I needed something to occupy my mind and my time. I looked around the shop at various art projects, stitch work, needlepoint, and paint-by-number kits. I had tried all these activities at different points of my life, but never finished any of them. I learned in rehab and in therapy that I had an issue with finishing things. I am inherently a perfectionist, and in therapy I discovered that once I had started using, I stopped tasks completely. I was afraid they wouldn't live up to the enormous expectations I had in my mind, so it was easier to make excuses as to why I never finished them.

That fear of imperfection kept me from finishing various things in my life. I barely graduated high school because I skipped so many classes and so many days that the administrators said I was too delinquent to attend graduation. The ceremony was seen as a privilege, and I didn't quite earn mine. After that I attempted to take some college-level classes, but stopped attending the classes midway through the semester because I just didn't feel like going. I was only twenty-two years old, but during my time in the workforce I'd had more than thirty-six jobs in almost as many fields: waitress, hostess, bartender, insurance claims adjuster, travel agent, receptionist, shampoo girl, medical assistant. You name it, and I had tried it—but never finished it. I would decide one day that I wanted to go to college and would start filling out applications, and then toss them aside to collect dust on my desk. Another day I would decide I wanted to be a flight attendant, call the agency, get the application, and tell everyone I was going to pursue this career, only to find the application months later sitting on top of the unfinished college applications. I was never committed to anything, so it was easy to abandon things. As I left for rehab, my former counselor looked at me and said, "Well, you are going to rehab for thirty days. Finish that." I did finish rehab, so that was my first completed task to date.

My new therapist was also big on getting me to finish at least one simple task. So as I stood in front of this wall of crafts, my eyes were drawn to a paint-by-number kit that showed two wolves and beautiful moonlit scenery. I picked it up and looked it over. It seemed easy enough; it came with the canvas labeled with numbers to show you where to paint each color, a plastic row of paints with coinciding numbers on them, and a cheap paintbrush with hard, plastic bristles. I decided if I was going to do this paint-by-number thing, I was going to take this work of art seriously, so I moved over to the paintbrush aisle to pick out a real paintbrush. I found a nice brush and went to the counter to pay for my new project. I didn't have a ton of money at the time, but my living expenses were zero under Matt's roof, I was able to collect a little bit of unemployment from my last job as a waitress, and my parents would send me some money every now and then.

When I arrived home, I pulled my purchase out of the bag and opened it with excitement, mainly because I was just happy to have something different to do with my time. I was fine when at therapy and meetings, but that only took up at the max three hours of my day. I was left to fill the other hours, which at this point was making me nutty. So with much anticipation, I set up a little painting studio in Matthew's living room, right in front of the TV, because it was close to 4:00 p.m. and *Oprah* was coming on. I began my hobby and became quite enthralled with this new activity.

I found painting very calming, which was exactly what I needed. I carefully filled in each numbered space with the corresponding paint color from the box. This became part of my daily routine. Wake up, drink coffee, avoid Matthew's advances, go to a meeting, on some days go to therapy, come home, eat lunch, paint and watch *Oprah*, wait for Matthew to come home, go to a meeting with him, usually just come home afterward, spend some time watching TV with his dad, and go to bed. The painting became the highlight of my daily life. Realizing that saddened me. I really was starting to feel as though I needed a job or some type of purpose.

By the way, I did finish the painting, and it was quite brilliant if I may say so myself. I framed that bad boy and gave it to my oldest brother, Jimmy, for a Christmas present. To this day, he still has it hanging on his wall. It is my one-piece ongoing art exhibit, and I am damn proud.

After finishing that artwork, and as a result of continual attendance in therapy, it was clear to me that I needed to get a job, get out of Matthew's house, and get out of the relationship, for that matter. I had been discussing the relationship in therapy, and, although my therapist never told me what to do, the day I mentioned it might be healthy for me to move out and end it, she was elated. It was becoming more and more difficult to pretend to be his girlfriend anyway. We never spent much time alone; we didn't interact as a couple in terms of kissing or having sex. Eventually, one night when he came into my room and attempted to slip into bed with me while his father was out, I had had enough, sat him down, and told him I was just not ready to be in a relationship—that I needed to focus on my recovery. I didn't have the heart to tell him that was only half true.

I just felt nothing for him sexually or romantically. It wasn't him—he was a sweetheart. It was me. There is a really good reason that counselors and others advise you to not be in a relationship during the first year of recovery. Everything is so raw and new, and the focus really needs to be on yourself and your program. However, this is not an easy concept for newcomers, especially us young ones, when we are finally feeling alive again in our bodies and hormones are raging. The sexual energy in a room full of young people in recovery can be a whole other type of intoxicating. It is quite surprising that on any given day you don't walk into a young people's meeting and see them all dry-humping each other like dogs in heat.

Matt did not take it very well when I told him, so I knew I needed to get the hell out of his house ASAP.

7

Sticking with Winners

By breaking up with Matt, I had just thrown my newfound routine and stability into upheaval. It was clear after dumping him that I had worn out my welcome and needed to move on. Even though I knew it was the right thing to do, I found myself very emotional after it all. I was sad for hurting him, but I also immediately missed the attention and "love" I thought I had received from him. I cried a lot about it—not so much over him but more for myself and the void I felt inside me. It was confusing, because I also found myself ecstatic about my new ability to vocalize my needs and actually follow through with them. So much change was going on inside me that I felt like I was on a daily roller coaster, and the ups and downs were making my head spin.

My sponsor, Tina, offered to let me live with her while I searched for an apartment. So I moved into her condo, closer to downtown

State College, which was where I wanted to be anyway. Everything was new—my room, the coffee maker, my surroundings, the neighborhood, everything. It freaked me out a bit because I was so used to my old routine. But it was a positive change, at least at first.

Tina's place was beautifully decorated and clean. Her mother was very wealthy. Her father had passed away, leaving her mom with a bundle, and she took care of Tina and paid most of her bills. Tina's condo had several bedrooms and a nice hot tub in the basement that I could retreat to when I needed it. It also offered me freedom from Matt. I felt as though I had more privacy and breathing room.

Tina hooked me up with a job with the company she was working for at the time. It was a biotech firm, a field I knew nothing about, but it was good pay. To help the company plan for a big conference, I was crafting correspondence, booking the conference locations, and having a blast. It felt so good to have purpose again and to be needed in a broader sense. It felt amazing to have a place to be each day, to be accountable to someone, and to be getting paid!

At Tina's house, though, I was aware I was still in someone else's space, so I was careful about my actions. I stayed in my room most of the time because I felt more ownership over that space. Plus, I was slowly noticing things about her that were red flags to me. She was often locked in her room most of the night. She rarely socialized with me. She seemed out of it a lot of the time. I couldn't quite put my finger on why my gut was telling me she may not have been the person she presented.

When I got into recovery, I had a whole new outlook on people and a naiveté that surprised me. I assumed everyone in recovery was just as honest and willing to work the program as I was. I assumed I could trust everyone in recovery. It was an assumption that I quickly learned was wrong. People from all walks of life come into the program, some for the right reasons and some for the wrong reasons, some who are sincere about getting help and some who aren't.

There are people who are mandated by the court to come into the rooms as part of their sentence, and you can usually spot them a mile away. They sit in the back of the room, they don't speak much, and they fly up to the meeting leader's chair to have their papers signed as soon as the meeting is over so they can get out of there. Not all of them are like this, of course. Some court-mandated attendees do get through the program and stick with it, but many just do their time and get their papers signed.

There are also those who come in and expound upon the text of their twelve-step fellowship, quoting every passage and page in the book like some kind of evangelist and trying to make everyone believe that because they memorized the book they are some type of recovery god. All the while they are hitting on the eighteen-year-old newcomer walking through the door or secretly gambling away all their money every Saturday night at a poker table.

Then there may be a girl who sits all the way in the in the back week after week, never saying a word. Everyone assumes she isn't getting it and will relapse any minute, until one day she does speak and says something incredibly profound and announces that she actually has five years of clean time.

As with any group of people, everything is not always what it seems. Recovery is a microcosm of society at large. So many of us come into the rooms of recovery having done some horrible, illegal, and unethical things, and yet overall most recovering people I've met are some of the most creative, loving, honest, and pure people I know. Many are still faking it just to make it. It took me a while to figure out who was who. I wasn't always as sharp as I wish I could have been. For example, I briefly dated a guy I thought was just as into recovery as I was, only to find that he enjoyed another compulsive disorder and would try to get me to watch porn every night. I befriended and became the sponsor of a younger girl who told me horrible sob stories that broke my heart. Later I would learn from her mother and her that she was a pathological and compulsive liar and the stories were all lies. I kept hearing people in the meetings say, "Stick with the winners," but my radar was still a little broken in that department and tended to guide me toward the familiar. I had made it a habit of sticking with the losers for so long.

Tina and I got along very well, but as I gained more time in recovery and my radar slowly began improving, it became clear to me that she wasn't as into the program as I had first suspected. As I became more involved in meetings and began to meet more people, I started to hear rumors that she was using. She was always one to talk the talk so well, but after a while I began to see through it. I think because we were living together, working together, and going to meetings together, I got to really see her day-to-day actions. She made unethical decisions with her mother's money, often making up stories about why she needed large sums of money, such as a car repair that wasn't real, and then she would go shopping. When she came home from work, we would chat for a little bit, but then she always locked herself in her room for the remainder of the night. I didn't think much of it initially, but eventually I began to have my own suspicions about her behavior.

One night after she locked herself in her bedroom and she thought I was in mine, I stood outside her door. I began to smell the all-too-familiar scent of marijuana wafting from her room. I knocked on the door and confronted her. She was all red-eyed and trying to say she was meditating and burning incense. I was no fool. I knew that smell, and she knew that I knew. I just walked away from her and went into my own room.

The next day I fired her as my sponsor and called my parents to let them know that I needed to get out of there right away. My parents were understanding immediately, and they began to treasure and protect my recovery as fiercely as I had. I was very hard on myself at first. Here I was, thinking I was making the right choices and doing the right things, but I was living with a sponsor who, instead of helping me with recovery, was lying to me and getting high right under my nose. I was so afraid of what others in the program would think of me. Would they think I was getting high as well? And I was ashamed at not realizing it sooner. I couldn't believe I hadn't realized she was high. I felt betrayed. And stupid. Once I had been able to spot an addict from a mile away, yet here this woman was, getting high right in the same house I was in, and I hadn't caught on. It was that naiveté again; I guess I just wanted to believe she wasn't using.

After that I found it difficult to sit in meetings and listen to Tina say all the right things and continue to stand up and get recovery chips, claiming that she had continuous recovery and clean time, which I and everyone else knew was bullshit. It wasn't my place to call her out in the meeting, nor was it anyone else's. After all, she had to live with her lies, and for anyone who has ever attempted recovery, that can be a hell unto itself. Coming into the rooms of any support group and making that first admission of having a problem tends to really put a damper on ever attempting to use again, because now you are aware it is a problem, and that acknowledgment echoes in your head and at least reduces if not ruins any high you attempt to achieve.

Tina's lies made me want to scream every time I heard her. And it hurt my feelings to know this person I once trusted enough to ask to be my sponsor was a hypocrite. So I avoided her and began to mix up my meetings so I was attending those I knew she wasn't attending. It was best for me to find new meetings and new people to hang around. It was how I started learning to stick with the winners. Unfortunately, Tina was no winner in the program, and I wasn't going to be a loser ever again.

Many years later, after I had been living in Harrisburg for a while, I got a call saying that her body had been found on the side of a highway just miles outside of State College. She had been shooting up and overdosed in her car. She died alone in her car on the side of a road with a needle sticking out of her arm.

8

NEW FRIENDS

MY PARENTS WERE VERY SUPPORTIVE OF MY NEW LIFE
and wanted nothing more than to help me. If I called and needed
something, they were there immediately. They mailed me care packages
to ensure I had basic needs, like beauty supplies, cigarettes, and
extra money to go out to eat or anytime I needed something. They
frequently sent me notes of encouragement that said how proud they
were of me. The cards reaffirmed that I was on the right track. They
made me lighten up when I opened and read them, and I proudly
displayed them.

When I caught Tina in her lie, I called my parents and told them
my living environment was no longer a safe place for me and my
recovery because my sponsor was using. My parents knew enough
about the program of recovery to know that the most important thing
is to avoid people, places, and things related to using. After talking,

we determined it was time for me to get my own apartment. This was something my parents had wanted me to do from the start. To this point in my life, I had never been on my own.

Before meeting my father, my stepmother was a fiercely independent woman. She had always provided for herself, and I knew she wanted me to experience that kind of freedom and security. My father was different. He always had been in a relationship, and up to that point, I had mirrored his actions. My parents had saved a good chunk from the insurance money left by my biological mother when she died three months before I went into rehab. Her death from breast cancer was one of the catalysts that got me into recovery. The pain of her loss was too much for me to bear, which helped me hit rock bottom quickly. My father and stepmother were smart about my inheritance when I got it after her death. Knowing that I was a mess and still using, they requested that I give them the money and allow them to dispense it to me as needed. For some reason I actually agreed to this, probably because I was such a mess, but also because I was making good enough money tending bar to feed my drug habit. So I didn't push the issue with them as long as they paid my bills and rent. Thanks to them, I ended up with a couple of thousand dollars left over. I used the money to find a cute little one-bedroom efficiency set in the woods about a mile from the Pennsylvania State University campus.

The apartment was an adorable space on the second floor of a two-story brick building in a large complex. Located off the main road and away from the more traditional student apartment complexes, it sat on a winding road nearly hidden in the woods. It was surrounded by trees, and a stream ran through my backyard. I could sit for hours on the wooden deck off my bedroom just reading, journaling, and enjoying my surroundings. It was quiet. The apartment complex catered to older students and families, and the managers screened the tenants carefully to try to avoid the typical party scene that would play out across the street at the more traditional student housing. It felt like an oasis, which was exactly what my soul needed at the time.

My parents loaded all of my former belongings into a U-Haul, brought along my cat that had been living with my brother, and drove up to help me move into my new apartment. I didn't have a ton of stuff left over—a bed, a dresser from my childhood (off-white with little pink flowers), a TV, a coffee table, and a black high-top kitchen table with two chairs that my mother had bought years ago and which I'd kept after her death. My parents and I went out and bought a futon so I had a place to sit and watch the small TV I had.

While we were moving things into my apartment, my father dragged my bed up the stairs into the tiny bedroom. As he hoisted it on top of the already existing box spring, my eyes were immediately drawn to a faint, red stain that covered a large portion of the mattress. I was transported back to that night—the night I hit my rock bottom, the night of my last drink and drug, the night I sliced away the flesh on my wrists in an attempt to kill myself. Tears flooded my eyes and my father became uncomfortable and said, "Oh, I forgot about that," and just like that, he flipped it over to its other white, clean side.

I stood there for a couple of minutes trying to regain my balance and focus on the present. He asked if I was okay. I just nodded. He mumbled something about the bed being so new he didn't want to throw it out, because I had just purchased it only three months prior to the incident, and blah, blah, blah. The "incident" is how we refer to what I did. I assured him it was fine and I was fine, and truly, I kind of was. The mattress, even white side up, would serve as yet another reminder for me, just like the soft scars on my wrists served as vivid reminders. At this early stage in my recovery, having as many reminders as possible was good. Anytime I would remotely think my old way of living wasn't that bad, I would look at those scars and they would scream a different story.

This activity is called "keeping it green" in the recovery community. It is about not shutting the door on our past, but allowing it to stay open enough for us to remember how bad it was at any given point in our addiction. Sometimes we call it "playing the tape all the way through." For example, if you think you want a drink, you play that scenario over in your head all the way through to its inevitable conclusion based on your past experiences. For me that would mean picking up a drink, then another and another, eventually craving cocaine and finding a dealer, staying out all night getting high, spending all my money, finding myself utterly desperate and depressed when the drugs are gone and the sun is shining in my face, disappointing my family, and losing my recovery time. I usually only get halfway through the scenario when it dawns on me that I am much better off not picking up that first drink.

That first drink—it's always all about the first one. You can't get to the other parts of that scenario without picking up the first drink, and that day, thank God I had enough tools from being in recovery for a while that I could talk myself out of the first drink. I also didn't have the desire to drink, really. That had been lifted from me very early in recovery. But I had the occasional craving and needed to deal with it just like everyone else.

At the time, I was reading a lot of recovery books, which really helped reinforce the principles of the program and gave me differing viewpoints on recovery. I wanted to learn as much as I could about recovery and how to continue on the path I was taking toward healing myself of my past wounds. So I began reading as much material as I could get my hands on. In meetings, there were often lots of books relating to recovery that brought me a deeper level of understanding of these concepts. I read these books whenever I felt like I needed an extra dose of recovery or when I was bored and found myself with time on my hands. In early recovery, keeping yourself busy and surrounded by the program is so important because it is easy to get sucked back into negative thoughts or to indulge the occasional self-pity or depression that naturally arises when making such major life changes.

I also began keeping a journal of all my thoughts, feelings, and daily occurrences. My therapist suggested it would be a good idea to maintain a daily journal to keep track of my progress and to help sort out my feelings on paper. I began to realize how helpful this tool was since I had a million things running through my head at all times. Fears, doubts, excitement—you name it, I was experiencing it, so it was good for me to spill the contents of my overflowing mind onto paper. Doing so helped defuse a lot of my fears and allowed me to process through emotions productively by writing them down, almost problem-solving or counseling myself while writing. Often I would start to write about a fear or a problem I was experiencing, and by the time I was done writing, I had figured it out on my own.

Some days I would just sit on my little deck and write about how peaceful the world around me seemed and about the vast contrast between my old life and my new. It helped me see the little things I had to be grateful for each day, which was especially helpful on those days when I was feeling particularly lonely or down on my luck. As great as things were going for me in my new town and new life, I still missed my family, my friends, and my old life—well, at least the good parts of my old life.

Because I needed to put space between myself and my former sponsor, I quit the job at the biotech firm. I was fortunate to have enough money to afford my apartment and live for a while without having to work full time. I knew I needed to start looking for a job soon, because the money wouldn't last forever and it would be good for me to have something to do during the day. Ironically, sometimes a lot of free time can be hard to manage. I began putting applications in at the mall at various retail stores and responded to an ad in the paper from a travel agency looking for a leisure travel agent. In my past I had worked as a corporate travel agent for a year, so I thought I might have a good shot at getting the job or at least an interview. Until then, I decided to focus on myself and my recovery.

I was making strides in therapy in that I was recognizing my relationship patterns and seeing them more clearly. I had broken up with Matt, but began immediately sleeping with another man in recovery. I always ran to the first person to pay me any attention. I knew it wasn't right, but I kept doing it. My therapist was trying to show me how I was still trying to fill the void inside me with something—in this case with sex and men. I was getting the idea, but slowly, because it didn't stop me from maintaining the relationship or the sexual activity. I was just so used to giving that part of myself over so freely that I thought it was normal, even though it didn't feel normal while doing it. It felt familiar, a feeling I confused with being okay. I was lonely in State College, and even though I was making some new great friends in the twelve-step program, it was still hard.

I was trying to connect with this new guy through sex, thinking that would bring us closer, but it proved to be wrong. I missed the people who really knew me, the ones I could call and not have to give a thirty-minute oral history of my life to before they would get what I was going through. I missed the connections I had with my old friends. At times I felt so alone, and it was hard to find people my own age who could relate to what I was going through. There are certainly not as many young people in the rooms of recovery as one would think, especially not many young females. Most of them, I guess, were still out exploring.

I did make friends with some of the older people in the rooms. I had always related to people much older than I was, so it worked for me, despite all evidence to the contrary in my past life. However, a handful of people around my age attended the meetings, and we began to form a young people's crew that was a lot of fun. We bonded quickly on the basis that we were all a little crazy, new to this whole recovery thing, lonely as hell, and craving friendship and attention. One other girl close to my age, Kate, was shorter than me and kind of socially awkward. She didn't say much and seemed to take to me immediately because I was much more talkative and brazen. If we were back in high school, I would have described her as the outcast type. She had super-long red hair, but the entire section underneath was shaved, which gave her a punk look when she pulled her hair up. She was a local, having grown up in State College, and was new to recovery just like me. We started hanging out often, going to meetings, going out for coffee, walking aimlessly around downtown together to kill time, and going to movies when we could afford it. We became inseparable even though we didn't have a whole lot in common. We shared a general loneliness and need for companionship that fueled our budding friendship. About five other young people slowly started joining us. We began to form this little gang, with our common denominator being that we hadn't a clue yet who the hell we were as individuals. As a group, though, we were able to feel a little closer to coming to that understanding.

Being with the group was fun. Every Friday night we would all hit a meeting together and then go to Denny's and spend hours there smoking and drinking enough coffee to keep us awake for the entire weekend. After reluctantly heading to our homes in the wee hours, we would all wake up by nine the next morning and stumble into a gratitude meeting with more coffee in hand and a whole different type of "hangover" than we were used to.

Another group of women, most of whom were lesbians, hung out together at the meetings. Immediately drawn to them, I began frequenting the meetings they went to and going out to eat with them too. A few weeks into getting to know them, I asked one of the women, Rose, an older, gentle woman in her early fifties with a spunky sense of humor, to be my sponsor. She agreed, and we began a great sponsor/sponsee relationship.

She made me call her every day and meet her at meetings each week, which I did. I loved how crass she was, and we connected on that level right away. She would often laugh in meetings at inappropriate times, and we would sit and giggle like high school kids. She got my warped sense of humor.

She was also patient with me, and when I would call her every day, sometimes with the same issue, she would guide me through the steps of recovery to help me understand how to resolve whatever it was. She encouraged me to read more and bought me my first daily devotional book that I loved immediately. It offered great lessons for each day of the year that clicked in my brain. Each morning, we would read our daily devotional and then talk about how it related to us. It helped us learn about each other. Rose was also just trying to come into her own sexuality, and I was drawn to her for that reason, too. I had yet to really sort out my sexual feelings toward women, even though I knew they still lingered within. I thought Rose could help me in that area too, and as we grew close, I began to confide in her about my feelings toward women.

I discovered it was nice to have a solid routine and people whom I began to rely on seeing daily. Better yet, people began to rely on seeing me. If for some reason I didn't show up at a meeting, my phone would ring and someone would be checking up on me to see that I was okay. The connection I was forming with these new friends gave me something I don't think I had ever really had—accountability. It began to offer me a different kind of stability, and, although it felt incredibly odd at times, it offered me a solace and more of that hope stuff I had begun to rely on as much as air.

As I was making these new friends, some of my old friends from the past began contacting me. I had tried to avoid them in the first couple of months while I focused on myself. It had been hammered into my head that old people, places, and things were to be avoided at all costs if I wanted to maintain my recovery. But I wasn't quite ready to let them go yet. I had especially missed my best friend Kathy. I figured that since now I was settled in my own place, had a solid sponsor, and was beginning to have a nice foundation in recovery, it couldn't hurt to reconnect with some old friends.

9

BEER PONG AND OTHER MISADVENTURES

ONE NIGHT IN MY FIRST YEAR OF RECOVERY, A BUNCH of my high school friends came into town to visit me and some of our other friends who were now attending Penn State University. These were girls I had hung out with in high school who were a year younger than me—not the girls in my grade I did my hard-core drug partying with—but we did do a ton of drinking together. They were really sweet girls and very supportive of my recovery. We all went to a fraternity party and were having a blast as everyone began playing beer pong. Beer pong is much like ping pong, except you place several cups filled with beer at each end of a table. The goal is to get your ball into another's cup, which that person then has to drink, all without using a paddle. It is one of those "get hammered in less than twenty minutes" games that occur in every frat house in town.

I never dreamed of attempting to actually play, so I stood off to the side and watched until one of my friends kept bugging me to play. The last thing I wanted to do was draw attention to myself and to the fact that I was the only one in the room *not* drinking, so I kept blowing her off and trying to get her to shut up. But she was adamant, and the owner of the house said something like "Yeah, why not? Come on, I think I have something here you can use instead of beer." He searched his nearly bare cabinet until his hand stumbled upon a big, round container of Lipton iced tea mix. Lucky me! He scraped the old tea mixture out of the tin can, mixed several cups of water with the iced tea mix, and set me up at the one end of the table. With all eyes on me, I wasn't about to say no, so I reluctantly gave in. I didn't want them to think I was a freak, and somehow I figured I could just blend into this fraternity life. So I took my position at the end of the table and began playing. With each toss of the ball, I felt excitement, like I was one of them. People were cheering me on and screaming my name and it felt exhilarating.

As it turned out, I was not very good at iced tea pong, and the other guy kept bouncing his ball into my little cups of tea. Each time the ball fell into my cup, I had to pick it up and slam back my cup of tea. It was super-sweet since he'd mixed in way too much of the old tea, but I kept slamming back the sugary, sandy drink, trying to keep my face from showing that it tasted like shit. I just wanted them to like me, and for once I wanted to not feel like a total outcast in this world.

After about twenty minutes of getting my ass kicked at this game and throwing back more cups of tea than I can remember, my stomach began to churn and a burp that had just a slight hint of vomit in it came bubbling up out of my throat. I realized quickly that I was about to get sick, threw my hand up over my mouth, and ran into the small bathroom in the hallway. I puked my brains out. Ice tea mix flew out of my throat like a rushing, fierce tide and sprayed the white toilet bowl like sand art. I was the only one in the room not drinking alcohol and still the first one to puke at the party—not much different from my old days of drinking. It was pathetic. As I sat there wiping my lips, I just had to laugh because here I was trying to be something I clearly was not anymore. And for what? Approval? Friendship? Acceptance? I should never have attempted to blend in. It all felt so stupid. This was not the place for me anymore, I realized. Just then I felt utter sadness in the pit of my stomach. "If this isn't who I am anymore, then who the hell am I?" I wondered.

A couple of days later, I talked about it in therapy and cried really hard because suddenly I didn't know who I was supposed to be. Everything in my life had changed, everything I once knew was shifting, and I had no clue where I fit in anymore. I didn't feel quite right with my old friends, and I was just learning how to feel comfortable with my new friends in recovery. Most importantly, I had no idea who I was.

My therapist had warned me about hanging out with old friends, saying I was putting myself in dangerous situations that would eventually lead me to use again if I wasn't careful. She was concerned about my need to keep my old friends. I knew she was right, but I wasn't totally ready to give them up yet. After all, I was twenty-two years old; what the hell was I supposed to be doing? Rose echoed my therapist's concerns, which gave me a double dose of guilt, but also helped to make me see that maybe once again my thinking was getting me into trouble. My therapist told me to make a list of all the things I enjoyed doing that didn't involve alcohol and to bring this list with me to our next session. Great—homework. That was something I definitely hadn't thought I would be doing at twenty-two.

But that weekend I had plans with my old high school friends again. We all decided to go to another party in town. My friends attempted to respect my recovery as best they could. They were protective of me because they knew everything I had been through, but they still wanted me to go out with them, so I did. Because I was doing so well in my recovery, none of us saw the harm in it. To them, I was still me, they wanted to hang out with me, and I wanted so badly to be around them as well. So I threw caution to the wind again and went.

Most of the people at the parties we went to weren't too fazed by my not drinking until they started getting loaded themselves. That is when all the questions and fascination would start. "Wow, you mean you don't drink at all? Like never?" People would slur questions into my face as though they were holding the Spanish Inquisition. I know most of them were well-meaning, but probably couldn't even imagine for a minute going out to a party or bar and not drinking, which was why they were fascinated with me. I was like a mythical creature they could not stop staring at, like a unicorn standing right there among them but with this strange power of *not* drinking. To others, though, I was the elephant in the room no one wanted to deal with. I symbolized what they could not achieve, and sometimes my presence brought out bitter resentment in people who didn't want to face their own demons.

On this night, the guy who was hosting the party wanted everyone to get in a circle and do a shot to him and his fraternity house. As everyone was moving into a circle, he was handing out shot glasses. I stepped back and tried as best I could to blend into the wallpaper behind me.

Of course, he noticed me while he made his way around filling the glasses and called me over to join the circle. I politely shook my head and said, "No thanks. I don't drink." He persisted. "Come on, it's just one shot, it won't kill ya," he said.

"No, thank you. I am really okay. You go ahead," I said, my voice shaking. I didn't like all the attention that was squarely focused on me. My friends looked at me wide-eyed, and one mouthed, "I'm sorry." But the host was not about to take no for an answer. He was a big dude and had been powerhouse drinking all night. "What the fuck do you mean, NO? This is my fucking house and my fucking party, and if I say you're doing a shot, you're doing a shot!"

"Seriously, I don't drink at all," I managed to say as I began to get scared. His eyes were getting wild, and I knew he was hammered. "What do you mean you don't drink? What the fuck is that? What are you doing at a frat party if you don't drink?" He moved toward me with the bottle in his hand. I began backing up toward the wall until I was stuck in a corner of the room. I just kept saying, "I don't drink," and "Just leave me alone." Then he lunged at me. His eyes were huge and filled with rage. As he screamed at me, drops of his alcohol-laced saliva hit my face. He kept berating me about not drinking, asking what kind of pussy I was that I didn't drink, and how dare I disrespect his house and his fraternity by not doing a shot with him? I could feel the weight of his body thrust against mine, and the wall behind me hit my back. He smelled like a brewery, and I turned my head to avoid his stench. Fear nailed my feet to the floor, and I couldn't move. He raised the bottle of booze and shook it. I was petrified it was going to spill out all over my head. I wished nothing more than for the wall behind me to open up and engulf me in the patterned wallpaper.

My two guy friends quickly came to my rescue. As they started pulling him away from me, a huge fight broke out. As soon as there was an opening, I ran over to my girlfriends and we fled the house as fast as we could. On our heels were our guy friends yelling for us to get in the car. As my ass hit the leather of the backseat, I was shaking violently. I fell into my friend's lap and burst into sobs. I had never had anyone treat me like that in recovery. I couldn't understand why this guy had such a visceral reaction to me. My friends assured me that he just was an asshole, but that was the last time they called me when they came to visit and the last time I ever went out to a frat party, or anywhere else, with any of them again.

10

FREAK

IN MY NEXT THERAPY SESSION, I SPOKE IN DEPTH WITH my therapist about the changes I was going to have to make in my life. I was so angry. I didn't want to be different, and I didn't want to be considered a freak, even if it was more in my head than in reality. She assured me I wasn't a freak and that life would be challenging at times, because no one can avoid alcohol altogether; it is a part of life and all over the place—in restaurants, in homes, at work parties. I needed to find a way to coexist with alcohol but to avoid places where drinking alcohol was the main purpose. We talked about my motives and how I always have to look at the reasons I am doing things. Why did I want to go somewhere? What was my goal for being at that party? Was it to fit in? To feel cool? I really had to look at the fact that those weren't acceptable reasons for me to put myself in harm's way. Before I could attempt to be who I always thought I should be or what others wanted me to be, first I had to figure out who I was. I felt trapped and lost somewhere between the party girl I used to be, whom everyone knew, and this new girl in recovery who felt emotionally naked and confused all the time.

I didn't feel the desire to drink or use even when I was out with my friends. I didn't feel pressured to drink. I thought those factors kept me immune to danger, or I did until the last party I went to with my old friends. I expressed to my therapist how incredibly scared I was that the bottle over my head was going to spill and the drops might have hit my lips or mouth. Would that have meant I had relapsed? My recovery was something I was beginning to treasure. Every time at a twelve-step meeting when I picked up a plastic chip for various lengths of time in recovery—sixty days, ninety days, 120 days—I felt proud, and I carried it around with me like a badge of honor. I began to realize how very precious this new life was to me and that I didn't want to tarnish it at all.

She asked me to pull out my homework, which I had anguished over all week. The assignment was one of the hardest tasks I had been given while in recovery. It was a self-exploration assignment. It felt stupid to write down all the things I liked to do that didn't involve alcohol. At first I sat there staring at the paper, and I felt as blank as the page. My head was empty as I tried to think of everything I liked to do before this recovery thing. I did *everything* high or with alcohol. There was rarely a time when I didn't use to enhance an event or experience. I figured I would start small—movies, I love movies. So I wrote:

1. Movies

A memory of dropping acid before going to see The Hand That Rocks the Cradle *came rushing back to mind. I remember I went to the bathroom right as I was peaking on my acid. I ended up in the stall for more than an hour, staring at the tiles on the walls as they slowly danced for me to the elevator music playing overhead. I missed half the movie.*

2. Bowling

Okay, bowling. Bowling was cool, but there were always bars at the bowling alleys, and, seriously, my score always improved after three or four beers.

Argh! Fuck, this was hard. I got frustrated as I realized that nothing I ever did was without alcohol or drugs. How was I supposed to even know what I liked when I was always fucked up? I crumbled up the piece of paper and threw it in the trash.

I ended up with no list and instead shared my frustrations with my therapist. She said it was normal to feel the way I felt, but suggested I really had to work hard at discovering what I like *now*. So she posed these questions to me:

1. *What does the recovering me like to do now?*

2. *What have I always wanted to do but have never done because drugs or alcohol got in the way?*

Those questions bounced around in my head as I left therapy that day. I thought of the peacefulness I felt while sitting on my deck reading and journaling. I liked that. I still loved movies and watched a ton at home without drinking, so I guessed I liked that. I enjoyed spending nights at Denny's with my new friends in recovery. I liked the true laughter that erupted from us all without any outside chemical influence. I still loved to listen to live music and to dance, but those things usually only happen in bars or at parties, and those bars and parties usually involve alcohol.

I still wasn't totally convinced that hanging out with my old friends wasn't the best idea. After all, these were people I had known half my life. But I was beginning to see that I was changing, and with every step of growth I took in recovery, I got further and further away from the friends I thought I had, and further away from the person I once was.

Sometimes I would go out and have a blast and enjoy just being clean and sober, but sometimes the nights would end with me feeling like a lost puppy. I would feel totally alienated from the people I thought I knew so well once they became engulfed in the party scene. I would often write in my journal about these times, as I did this one night while caught at a party and feeling my skin begin to crawl.

Sometimes I feel so incredibly alone in my own skin and in this world that the isolation of being a recovering addict is painfully deafening in a room full of laughing social drinkers enjoying petty conversations and flirting. I feel like in an instant the room stops and swirls around me, and they all stop and stare at the freak who can't compare. At the girl who took it too far and now lives in shame beyond repair. She gets all dolled up and looks the part, but when it comes down to it she can't cut the rug up like you do after four or five fuzzy navels.

Her insecurities shine on her forehead and her confidence falls to the floor in beads of sweat from her lower back, releasing all that she thought she was, only in a moment uncovering her weakness and exposing her darkness to a room full of oblivious drunkards. She desperately looks into the eyes of the strangers who have formed around her, who were in an instant transformed by the elixir of the evil that once tempted her, turning everyone from friend to foe. Her breath catches as she sees the confusion in her loved ones' eyes because what is staring back at her is a total surprise. She can't handle this person who is suddenly standing before her, small, wilted. She looks unfamiliar against the backdrop of the strength you know her day-to-day shell to be. And you can't move, like your feet are trapped in a vise that contorts. Your voice shakes coming up your throat and out of your mouth as you try to explain that today is just one of those days I once mentioned to you that I could possibly have while trying to be "normal." Some days it is so foreign, the space between the old life and the new one, that I get so lost in a tunnel of what-ifs and once-was's that I can't see the water filling up around my feet as it quickly engulfs me and I find myself drowning in the probability that you won't really like me once you really see me.

Some nights were hard, but the more recovery I gathered, the more I learned that going out to bars and trying to act *as if* was not only *not* in my best interest, it could result in my own relapse. In recovery, you have to be vigilant about your disease. You have to sometimes place your needs and recovery above everything and everyone else. This can seem incredibly confusing and selfish to those not in recovery, but for those of us in recovery, it seriously means life or death. However, like a good addict by nature, I would have to learn this lesson by trial and error—over and over again.

II

SUPERHERO

AT THIS EARLY STAGE OF MY RECOVERY, WITH NOT EVEN a year under my belt, I still wanted to be around my friends and also my family, even though I had chosen to move away and knew it was not a good idea. I needed to feel connected to them, and being four hours away was really hard. Both of my brothers were living in their own addiction at that time, and I hoped that by going home I could show them that recovery was an option and a good one. I thought I could save them. I was misguided.

I would go home and visit my brother Brian who was living in a one-bedroom apartment in the same complex where my brother Jimmy was living with his girlfriend and their daughter, Cheyanne.

Brian was in rough shape. I remember going to his apartment one Saturday morning and knocking on the door. I banged loudly and heard nothing. I kept banging, and finally I heard a rumble and my brother faintly grunting. As he opened the door, I could see he was shirtless but wearing a pair of dirty jeans. His hair was matted and messy and he was squinting hard at the sun that had suddenly flooded the dark apartment and his vacant eyes. He pulled his head down to avoid the sun and eye contact, and he motioned me in through the door. As I walked in, the stench of stale beer and cigarettes filled my now-flaring nostrils. I waded through the mess of clothing, crushed beer cans, and random trash cluttered around my feet as I stepped toward the couch. A beat-up love seat sat on one side of the room, and a mismatched, beat-up couch had been pushed against the wall. In between, a worn-out coffee table was littered with cigarette butts and ashes, beer cans, a little pile of pot seeds, and an overflowing ashtray.

I sat down and my skin began to crawl from the smell and environment. My mind flew back to how many times I had allowed myself to fester in environments similar to this—the all-night crack binges, the hangovers, and the horrible mornings that followed. I pulled out my cigarettes, fired one up as fast as I could, and handed my brother one too. I lit my brother's cigarette, sat back, and took in the sight of my brother before me. His face was broken out with angry, pus-infected pimples scattered all over his forehead, cheeks, and neck. Just from that I knew he was doing a lot of coke. I remembered how my face would break out, and a shiver went up my spine. I tried to make idle chitchat with him, talking about my new apartment and how great the recovering community was in State College. He wasn't really hearing me; he just looked over and asked me if he could borrow twenty bucks. He was supposed to have been paid at the bar where he was working, but they stiffed him … blah blah. I knew he was handing me the standard line of bullshit I had been so familiar with giving only months before, but I didn't let on that I knew he was full of shit. Instead I felt nothing but pity and sadness for him. His hopelessness was palpable. I wanted nothing more than for him to see how well I was doing and to begin to understand that he, too, could be okay.

He said he hadn't really been eating much because he didn't have money, and I could tell that was true. My brother had always been skinny. When we were little, everyone in our neighborhood called him "Ethiopian," because no matter how much he ate, he always seemed to weigh about as much as a sack of groceries. Today I could see his rib cage was just a little more pronounced, his stomach more concave than usual. He saw me looking at him. I pushed out a little laugh and said, "Ethiopian," and I saw a glimmer of light flash across his eyes, a brief recognition and connection to our past—our uninhibited, unencumbered childhood before addiction took charge of it all. He laughed and said, "Yeah, whatever, Keenifer," a nickname I had always loathed because when I was a child my brothers taunted me unmercifully with it until I cried. Lately I had come to love it, because as I grew into an adult, it became one of those playful things that embodied everything about innocence. It's one of those words that can send me into a tailspin of memories of pigtails, ice cream trucks, and all things hopeful and lingering from my days as a little girl.

Brian made a joke about going into the store and buying four packages of ramen noodles because they were only about twenty cents a package. Something about the image of him walking up to the cashier and handing over a pocketful of spare change for what would be a week's worth of food was too much for me to bear, and my heart sank as sadness flooded me.

I pushed the pain down and swiftly began speaking about how great rehab was, how my new life in State College was amazing, how meetings aren't that bad, that cool people were there, and that I thought he should come and stay with me for a little bit. His eyes dropped to the floor and he nodded his head, agreeing, "Yeah, I am sure it's great. Maybe sometime I will visit."

I wanted nothing more than to connect with him, for him to see how well I was and to want what I had. If I could have physically force-fed my recovery down his starving throat, I would have sat there all day spooning it to him. But he didn't want to hear it; he wasn't hearing me at all. I was just external chatter bouncing off him like background noise in a bar. I realized that no matter how much I loved him, there would be no penetrating the brick wall of denial that enclosed him until he was ready to start lifting up the bricks and seeing beyond it himself.

His blank, dark eyes were off in another place, a place of desperation that was beyond my reach at this point. I recognized that look, and I understood the denial and despair that went along with it. Reluctantly, I also realized I was no match for his disease that day. I reached into my wallet and handed him a twenty-dollar bill. He took it without meeting my eyes and said, "Thanks, man. You have no idea how much this will help." Then he jumped up and said he had to be at the bar to paint; he wanted to make sure he was there so he could finish the job and maybe get paid and then he would pay me back. I responded, "Yeah, whatever. It doesn't matter. Whenever you can," knowing I would never see that twenty dollars again and wishing against all odds that he would use it for food instead of beer and dope.

Visiting Jimmy wasn't much better, except the house was cleaner and his daughter, my little Cheyanne, was there for me to play with. I loved her and cherished every minute I could spend with her. Something in her big brown eyes, when they looked up into mine, made me feel like I was seeing myself. Whenever she was fussy or crying, all I had to do was scoop her up in my arms and she would gently release her tensed-up body against mine, slowly rest her little head on my shoulder, and quiet down. I would sometimes rock her to sleep and end up putting myself into a peaceful, calming, meditative state for hours. There really is no feeling quite like having a baby asleep in your arms. It is like God's perfection right there for you to hold, feel, and smell. It is brilliant!

Jimmy was still tending bar at the place I used to frequent— the same one where Brian was supposedly painting. It was a decent nightclub, but to me it held memories of many drunken, high, rough nights out on the town. It was a place I never wanted to frequent again, so I didn't go there to visit him. Instead I visited his apartment, but I could tell his life was just as chaotic as it always was.

My parents had told me about the fights he and his girlfriend got into, and she would call me screaming about what an asshole he was and how she was going to leave him. It was total drama—drama in which I normally would have been cast in the supporting role. But today the drama just drained me of all energy. I couldn't stand listening to it because it sucked the life out of me. It made me extremely grateful that my life, while still unknown and frustrating at times, was no longer a drama fest. Even though I was still fighting the idea that I could hang out with my old friends, the usual drama that came with all that was subdued by my lack of participation in the partying.

Eventually I stopped driving home every weekend to see my brothers. It was pretty obvious I could do nothing to help them. I saw my niece as often as I could, usually while my parents were caring for her, so I wasn't forced to walk into the sadness and destruction my brothers' lives had become.

I had really thought I could save them, as though my cape of recovery swinging behind me would be a sure signal to them of hope and a chance for a different life. But I slowly realized I just had to love them, pray for them, and let them go. I could still be an example for them, but not an in-your-face example. I knew the more I tried to hang out with them in their element, the more dangerous it would be for me. It's like a saying they have in the rooms of recovery: "If you sit in a barber shop long enough, you are bound to get a haircut."

12

No Really Means No

I HAD BEEN LIVING IN MY NEW APARTMENT FOR A
couple months and still wasn't dating anyone. I was taking a break after
Matthew, as the people in the program had suggested. The first time
my friend Kathy came from Allentown to visit me in State College, I
was so excited. Although we maintained our friendship with almost
daily phone calls, she hadn't been to see me in State College once,
so I felt I had been making all the effort by going home to visit her.
She surprised me for my birthday with tickets to see Pearl Jam, who
were performing about an hour from State College. I was ecstatic and
couldn't wait for her to come. She and her sister Jen were driving up on
Friday and were staying all weekend. The concert was on Sunday, and
they were going to leave right afterward.

Kathy and Jen arrived close to 6:00 p.m. that Friday. As they
unpacked, I saw Kathy pull out a big bottle of vodka. She asked if it

was okay to put it in my freezer. Seeing the bottle made me a shiver a bit, but I didn't have any craving to drink it, so I shrugged and said, "Sure." She still drank heavily, and when I came home to Allentown and we hung out, my recovery wasn't something she ever considered when slamming back her shots. With the alcohol out of sight, we began catching up and talking about how excited we were to see the concert. We were blaring Pearl Jam songs in preparation. My excitement was growing since I had never seen Pearl Jam live before. I loved going to concerts and had all my life. In fact, I had just gone with my brother Brian to see the Further Festival, which was the Grateful Dead minus Jerry Garcia, and I was amazed at how much better the music actually sounded when I wasn't on anything.

We were heading to a party that night held by some of Kathy's Allentown friends who were going to school in State College. I was slightly apprehensive about going to a party. Kathy did several preparation shots of vodka, and then we were on our way to the party. I drove her car because I was the only one not drinking. The party was in full swing when we pulled up to the little ranch house. People had spilled out onto the front lawn and were scattered on the side of the house and sitting on the curb, drinking and smoking. The sight was commonplace in downtown State College on the weekends, with house parties everywhere and people stumbling all over town drunk off their asses. No cops seemed to notice, or if they did, they simply looked the other way.

The house was packed and music was blaring as we navigated our way through the front door and into the kitchen where Kathy's friends were. A blue plastic container in the corner of the room held a big silver keg. I stared at it for a moment as someone tapped off a fresh beer. It immediately sent me back to my drinking days. I could smell the foam that was sliding off the side of the plastic cup. I felt the weight of the cup being placed in my hands as it had been so many times before. I could taste the bitter rush of that first sip as it awakened every taste bud in my mouth. I didn't realize I had been staring at the keg while trapped by these memories until a guy with a beer in hand called out, asking me if I wanted one. I must have looked like a moron as I briskly shook my head no. I was trying more to shake the memories free from my head than decline the beer, though it accomplished both. The guy turned around to engage another partygoer as I continued to shake my head a bit to get rid of the last of my thoughts. I calmly told myself, "I am in recovery now and that is not my life anymore." It worked, and I regained my footing enough to move into the living room.

I made small talk with some people and mingled for a while. Kathy was sitting on the couch getting stoned with a guy friend of hers whom she liked to hook up with every now and then when they were fucked up. She waved me over and introduced me to his friend Ted, a hippie dude with long, dirty blonde hair and an adorable smile that he flashed my way as he held out his hand to shake mine. He asked me to sit down with him, and I agreed. We started bullshitting, and he asked how Kathy and I knew each other as the pot pipe that Kathy was hitting began making its way over to my side of the room. Ted grabbed it and offered it to me. I looked at it momentarily as a little stream of white smoked danced above the silver bowl, and I said, "No, I don't get high anymore." He cocked his head back and gave me an inquisitive look. I simply answered, "I used to drink and get high a lot, too much in fact, and I recently got into recovery." He gazed at me as he took a huge hit off the pipe. While blowing it out his mouth, he nodded his head up and down as if in approval and said, "Right on, dude. I got a cousin who's in recovery. That is cool. Good for you." And just like that, Ted accepted my recovery as he blew out his hit of the pipe.

It felt good to have someone be so nonjudgmental of me, and suddenly I felt happy. I must have had some dumb-ass smile on my face because Kathy started cracking up at me, which sent the entire room into giggles. I laughed along with them, even though my reasons for laughing were clearly different. It felt good to laugh real laughter and not the pot-induced laughter they had. It also made me feel as though I fit in, even if just for a moment—as though I wasn't this outcast trying to blend into an environment that I really had no business being in anymore.

The party began to thin out. Kathy had disappeared somewhere with her guy friend. I hadn't seen her sister in hours. I was sitting on the couch with Ted, talking away a mile a minute. We were asking each other everything from what his major was to how I got to State College. I didn't share a lot with him. I didn't tell him how bad my drinking and drugging had been or about rehab or anything. I didn't feel totally comfortable with him, and I wasn't about to start throwing my life experiences at him. I also didn't want to reveal too much for fear it would scare him away. I liked him; he was sweet and had that killer smile that made me feel warm every time he flashed it my way.

It was getting really late, and Ted caught me letting out a huge yawn. He mentioned needing to crash soon himself. We went to search for Kathy or Jen. Ted said he figured Kathy was in his roommate's bedroom, and as he cracked open the door, sure enough, there they were, lying in bed together making out. I asked her when she would be ready to go because I was tired. She looked over at me with wide eyes and said that she was planning to stay over. I sighed and asked where her sister went so we could go home. She said that she had given Jen her keys and let her take the car back to my house about an hour earlier. She muffled an apology, saying that I had been busy talking with Ted and she didn't think I would mind staying over. She said we would call Jen in the morning to pick us up.

I was pissed. I couldn't believe she gave Jen the car and that she left us there. I closed the door, since Kathy had returned to her making-out session again. Ted shrugged and said, "You can crash with me," and flashed me a sly, shit-eating grin. I was flattered by his interest and thought he was a really sweet guy. After all, we had just sat on the couch and talked for hours without him so much as touching me, so I thought it might be innocent enough to crash there, but I was nervous as hell. I just nodded and said, "Okay." He led me to his room across the hall and turned a light on low. The room was tiny, with a dresser, a desk, and his twin bed pressed up against the length of the wall. There was a little window above the side of the bed. He sat down and began getting undressed, and I felt the heat rise in my face. I began wondering what the hell to do. I slowly took my shoes off and asked him if he had a T-shirt and boxers. He handed them to me, switched off the light, and climbed into bed. I was left in the dark in some guy's room with his boxers and T-shirt in my hand. I slowly got undressed, my head swimming with a million and one different scenarios of what might possibly happen once I slipped into his bed.

I had spent my entire sex-filled years lying under men, giving in out of some assumed responsibility I had built within me for fear that if I didn't they would take advantage of me or hurt me. I didn't really know what it was like to want to have sex and then act on it while not using. Matthew and I had only tried to have sex a couple of times, and when we tried it didn't feel right. But maybe that was just Matthew, I thought.

I quickly crawled into bed and rolled over to my side with my back facing Ted. He rolled over and threw his arm around me, his hands quickly beginning to fondle my body. He began to kiss the back of my neck and moved my hair away to access my shivering skin. I could feel him get hard up against my back, and I froze in total fear. I didn't know what to do, how to handle this, so I just lay there while he kept kissing my back and running his hands over my body. It felt wrong, but still I just lay there. After a few minutes, he tugged on my shoulder and rolled me over and quickly pushed himself on top of me. It was dark, so I am sure he didn't see the pure fear in my eyes. He leaned down and kissed me, and that felt okay. I kissed him back a while, and before I knew it, his hand had slipped between us. He pulled his penis out and attempted to wriggle his boxers off of me. My head was screaming, "NO! NO! I don't want to do this. I don't know this guy. NO!" But of course, nothing came out of my mouth. As usual, it all stayed in my head—my strength, my voice, my choice was all in my mind.

He pushed himself inside me and began to thrust as my head swam with memories of every sexual encounter I had ever had, good and mostly bad. They were spiraling around in my head like a tornado, and I began to panic. A rush of strength came to me from somewhere in the whirlwind of memories and I yelled, "NO!" out loud. Ted stopped and looked down at me with a puzzled look on his face. "What? Are you okay?" he asked in a panicky voice. I replied, "No, actually I am not. Can you please stop? I don't want to do this." My voice was shaking but strong. And just like that, Ted rolled off me and curled up next to me, trying to stare into my eyes, although it was too dark to see.

I couldn't believe what had just come out of my mouth. I felt a rush of relief and fear come over me all at once. I didn't know what he would do, and I didn't want him to think I was a freak, but something about the whole experience felt so wrong that I couldn't remain silent. Silent was how I had been for so many years, for so many men and so many sexual encounters. He gently reached his hand across my forehead, swiping my hair off my face, and asked if I was okay. I felt embarrassed and proud as I responded yes and thanked him for stopping. "Dude, I would never do anything you didn't want me to. I'm not like that," he replied. He scooped me up in his arms and fell asleep. I lay there in his arms in amazement, not just at what I had just done and said but also at his response. All these years, I had been so fearful to assert myself with men because of my past sexual abuse and my incredible insecurities about wanting and needing approval, that I had never realized I do have a choice in this whole sex thing.

13

LETTING GO

SATURDAY MORNING I'D AWAKENED TO KATHY knocking on the door saying her sister Jen was there to pick us up. I got out of bed with Ted still half-asleep next to me. I bent down and kissed his cheek, whispered "thank you," and left. He didn't know it, but he had just given me a really important lesson.

We were supposed to go out that night to a local bar to see a band play. Kathy pulled the liquor bottle out of the freezer and poured herself and her sister drinks in preparation for us going out. She then grabbed a lemon out of the cooler she had brought and began slicing it. I knew what was about to transpire. Kathy would start throwing back shots as she always did and would get out-of-hand loaded in no time. That is exactly what she did, but on this night in particular, it was as if she were on a whole different kind of roll. She did more shots than I had ever seen her do.

I was starting to get annoyed with Kathy and her behavior. About three hours and who-knows-how-many shots later, we were ready to head out to the bar. Kathy was stumbling all over the place and was drunker than I had seen her in a long time. I drove us to the bar, and she was slurring and singing her head off out the window. We got to the bar, one in State College that I had never been to before, because why would I have been there? And I wasn't sure what I was doing there on this particular night except that this was what I had always done with Kathy. We never went to movies or just hung out playing games or any of the things that were beginning to occupy my days and nights now. Kathy, already drunk out of her mind, bellied up to the bar the minute we walked in and ordered another shot and a beer. I sat down next to her and lit up a cigarette. I ordered a diet soda and slowly scanned the crowd. The place was pretty packed with tons of frat boys and sorority chicks, the band was in full swing, and the whole scene reminded me of my old days. The bar stool felt shaky under my ass, and I really didn't want to be there. Kathy had ordered a couple more shots for her and Jen. She slammed back her shot, got up, and stumbled her way to the bathroom.

The bartender looked at me and watched cautiously as Kathy crawled back from the bathroom and slid onto her bar stool, almost missing it altogether and slouching over into my lap in a fit of giggles and nasty burps. She pulled herself to the bar and yelled at the bartender to give her another shot. The bartender looked at her in familiar disgust and motioned to me that he was cutting Kathy off. Kathy attempted to bring her body into alignment and got belligerent, slurring obscenities at him. Midway through "Get me a fucking drink," Kathy crashed to the floor. I looked down and saw her feet all mangled and her hair all over her face. She was laughing hysterically. The bartender motioned to the bouncers, and before I could reach her they grabbed her under each arm, hoisted her up, and swiftly glided her drunken ass out of the bar. I quickly grabbed her sister, and we took over for the bouncers outside the club. I was so embarrassed, just shaking my head at the bouncers and apologizing as Jen and I struggled to get Kathy to the car. We threw her in the back seat, where she continued laughing and rambling on about how the bartender was an asshole and how she wanted to go back there and kick his ass.

Somehow we managed to get Kathy out of the car and up the flight of stairs into my apartment. We dumped her now half-lifeless body onto my bed, where she rolled over and passed out. I was drained and disgusted. I pulled out the couch and made a bed for Jen while making one for myself on the floor. This whole night had been a disaster; in fact, the whole weekend was becoming too much. My connection and friendship with Kathy was being strained more and more every time we hung out. We just weren't in the same places in our lives anymore, and the drunken "let's get ripped and out-of-hand" bar scene no longer sat well with me. I fell asleep sadly knowing that things between Kathy and me were about to really change. At least we had the Pearl Jam concert to look forward to the next day.

I woke up to Kathy's raspy voice talking to someone on the phone. I heard her crying and saying that she was out of control and she didn't know what to do. I pretended to be asleep until she came out of the room fully dressed with her bag in hand. She shook Jen awake and said good morning to me. Jen rubbed her eyes, looked at Kathy, confused, and asked what she was doing. Kathy looked over at me and said, "Sorry, kid, I was messed up last night. I'm just gonna head home. Sorry about the concert. Here are the tickets if you still want to go." Disappointment and anger flooded me as I looked at her and shook my head. "Whatever, dude. Drive safely," I said as I passed her and went to the kitchen to make coffee.

I was so hurt and so pissed off. I couldn't believe she was just going to leave and not go to the concert she promised me for my birthday, which we had planned for months and that I was so excited to see. My blood began to boil, but when I opened my mouth to say something, nothing came out. Kathy's eyes were bloodshot, and she looked so pathetic. My anger quickly dissolved into pity. I knew that look. I knew she was badly hung over and feeling like death. I knew my saying anything would have just made her feel worse. So I helped her load the car and waved as she and Jen pulled out of my driveway.

I knew our friendship was over. There was no longer any substance to the relationship, and I began to wonder if there ever had been. I had moved past her and past that lifestyle. Instead of going to the concert, I cried all day as I grieved for the friendship and my loss of her in my life. Everything I once knew as truth was different. Everyone I once knew as my family and friends was different, and it was incredibly painful. I felt very alone and incredibly sad. I had to fully understand that I had nothing in common with the majority of the people from my past, and that was a crushing revelation. These were the people who made up my history, my life—the ones I thought knew me the best. And now I had to face the reality that without the partying, there wasn't a whole lot of substance to most of my friendships.

That weekend was the first time in recovery that I was truly and deeply disappointed and hurt by someone I was so close to. I had to be careful how I dealt with these emotions, because in the past this was the stuff that used to cause me to pick up a drink or drug.

I went to therapy the next day and shared my whole weekend and the mess it had been. I spoke about Ted, and how I almost made the same mistakes that I always made with men, but that something stopped me, and somehow for the first time in my life, the loud "No!" in my head actually came out of my mouth. And, surprisingly to me, he respected that and left me alone. I talked about Kathy and the conclusions I had come to about our friendship. My therapist just sat in silent agreement; these conclusions that were new to me were things she knew already. The beauty of therapy is that you have to figure things out on your own.

My therapist could have easily judged me and told me that what I was doing was dangerous and that I put my recovery at risk every time I walked into a bar or a party. But instead, she let me make mistakes and come to my own conclusions, and then she gently led me to deeper understanding of myself and my actions by listening and providing positive feedback. Because of this, I never felt that I had to hide anything from her. I didn't keep any secrets because I knew she wouldn't judge my actions or try to scold me for my sometimes ridiculous behavior. She let me be human, which was exactly what I needed.

I would just let it rip in her office, no filter on, rambling all over myself with my newfound dialect. I was so liberated by being able to express myself freely for the first time; my inner thoughts, fears, and experiences all spilled out at the feet of my very capable and, surely at times, amused therapist.

After that weekend I didn't hear from Kathy again, and my visits home to Allentown came to a grinding halt. I knew I had to really let go of *all* of my past and simply start my new life in State College. I still went home to see my parents on holidays and they came to visit me, but there was no more trying to save my brothers or trying to fix my friends. I finally fully accepted that I was no longer one of them and that trying to masquerade around with them only brought danger and heartache for me.

14

No Filter

I WENT HOME TO MY APARTMENT AFTER THERAPY, STILL trying to wrap my mind around all the events of the weekend. I had so many feelings swimming around in my head and no real method to sort them all out. The thing about early recovery was that everything was excruciatingly real, and feelings came in and out of me like a freight train with no warning and no schedule. I was slowly learning how to feel and how to identify my feelings and how to appropriately process them, but it was a daily, sometimes minute-by-minute struggle.

One day, for example, I had the brilliant idea of buying this herbal supplement called ginkgo biloba, because I had heard that it aided memory. In early recovery, I found myself extremely forgetful and sometimes had a hard time concentrating on one task for a long time. From speaking to my therapist, I knew this was common for people newly in recovery, especially for those of us who used to smoke pot like cigarettes. It takes time for memory and cognitive function to totally return. At this point, I was constantly forgetting my car keys. I would often lock myself out of my apartment and have to go the main office to ask maintenance to let me in.

After the fifth time this happened, I decided to take action and went to the store and bought a bottle of ginkgo biloba. I took the prescribed dose, and after an hour, I started feeling really weird—almost like I was tripping on acid. My pulse quickened suddenly and everything around me became enhanced. The room felt like it was closing in on me and my chest tightened as I began gasping for air. I thought I was having an allergic reaction to the pills. I began to freak out and was so scared. I felt like I had used, like I had relapsed, and that feeling was pushing me over the edge. I pulled out the phone book, looked up poison control, and dialed frantically.

The staff person answered, and I rambled into the phone about how I had taken the pill for memory, explained how I was feeling, and at the end threw in that I was in recovery from drugs and alcohol. She listened patiently, and when I was done she calmly asked me what drugs I used to do. When I answered, "Cocaine," she almost chuckled. She told me this was a common reaction for someone who used to abuse amphetamines. The way ginkgo works in the body is to help maintain blood vessels, thereby improving blood flow to the brain and extremities, which can re-create the sensation of being high. I wasn't the first to call with a similar reaction, which made me feel a little less anxious and stupid. She instructed me to make myself puke to get it out of my system if I didn't like the feeling.

I thanked her, hung up the phone, quickly ran to the bathroom, stuck my toothbrush down my throat, and puked. I sat on the bathroom floor for a while, shaken up by the experience. Here I was, hugging the porcelain god once again, but thankfully for a whole other reason. I still felt horrible, as though I had done something to jeopardize my recovery—and that paralyzed me. It was late, too late to call Rose, so I called one of my new recovery friends and told him what I had done. He laughed, and we talked for a while as he assured me my recovery was intact and fine. It is a learning process, and I just hit a little stumbling block. I tried to laugh it off because certainly there was some humor to be found in it. I decided it was better to forget my keys occasionally than to deal with that feeling ever again, so I threw the bottle away.

I hadn't wanted to use since I went to rehab; however, I had thought about escaping because sometimes it was all too overwhelming to deal with.

This night was the first night I started to think about getting high again. I had just started working at the travel agency and decided to call in for a day off the next day, because when I woke up I was still shaken up. I wanted to scream like a fitful child in a state of rage—in many ways that is what I was. I picked up my journal and was shocked by what I wrote:

> The pain, pain won't go away.
>
> There is only one thing I know, it's the only way.
>
> You say you got some and I'll be by your side.
>
> With it all my pain and anger I can hide.
>
> Just one hit I tell myself
>
> and we'll put the can back on the shelf.
>
> 200 bucks
>
> and five hours later, I'm feeling that stiff junkie rush
>
> and I've gotta have more.
>
> Baby, baby, where can we score?
>
> It's 4:00 a.m. and I want more.
>
> Can't stop now and can't have fun,
>
> You say she's asleep

but I don't care because if you're dealing to me

you better know it's a twenty-four-hour job

and I'll be your best client.

Just need a little advance to take me higher.

See I need it now and I will pay you later.

Cause the pain I'm feeling now don't get any greater.

Just one more hit and I'll be fine.

If that's all you got then I will settle for a line.

I was a child who never learned how to deal, how to feel, and how to get through anything without detaching from it, escaping from it, or medicating it in some way. Surges of emotion ripped through me like electrical currents, and I feared at times that if I opened my mouth and spoke, I would shoot bolts of lightning directly into the path of whoever was there. I didn't know how to speak my truth yet in a productive manner. Writing helped. It was always a great way for me to address the stuff that was flying around in my mind and place those thoughts safely outside my head into a journal. In recovery, we were told to expose our disease as often as it comes up. The reality of actually saying my thoughts out loud or seeing them on paper often took the power out of them and helped me to realize it is okay to have these thoughts. I am an addict, and therefore will most likely have thoughts like these forever. My recovery depends upon *what I do* with those thoughts in the moment. So I began exposing my disease every chance I could get—verbally and in writing.

Therapy and meetings were great places for me to begin to open my mouth and speak about the goings-on inside my cluttered head. The meetings helped me begin to compartmentalize all the baggage of my past, but they were only a couple of hours a week. I still had the other twenty-two-odd hours in the day to deal with, so I would write. I started to feel as though I had the vocal form of Tourette syndrome, because some of the shit that would fly out of my mouth was beyond inappropriate. I had no emotional or verbal filter. Whatever came to my mind somehow came out of my mouth and often hung in the air like a really bad fart.

My sponsor Rose would just laugh at me and assure me that it would pass, that I would begin to figure out how to grasp my emotions and become able to share them appropriately. She reminded me it was all about progress, not perfection, and that as I grew healthier I wouldn't immediately want to share every random thought or feeling that entered my body with everyone around me. I was a little uncertain, since I had gone from one extreme to another, which is quite common in early recovery. I went from never sharing anything or expressing myself to verbally and emotionally vomiting all over everyone around me. How unpleasant for them.

So there I was, home from therapy with all these realizations of who I was and who I was becoming. I ran a hot bath and disrobed as I thought about Ted and Kathy. I knew there was great meaning in everything that had happened over the weekend, but I just couldn't shake it all up in my head enough for it to fall into place. I felt anxious and utterly drained. I lit a bunch of candles and turned on some peaceful music as I slipped my aching body into the warm bubbles. Tension slowly released from my shoulders, and my head started to unwind a bit.

I thought about Ted as my hands began to slowly trace my body, trying to find some connection to it. I realized that I didn't know my own body; I had never really understood it or loved it in any way. I had used it, abused it, and detached from it so many times that I was unsure of its soft and curvy terrain. I didn't understand sex; I never had a healthy place to start understanding my own sexuality, other than starting with my body, my hands, and my own touch. I began gliding my hands over my supple breasts and felt my nipples get hard under the pressure of my thumb. I'd never really enjoyed anyone touching my breasts, and this sudden surge of excitement caught me off guard, but I gave into it as my body sank deeper into the steaming water. I let my hand travel farther and allowed the multiple sensations to overcome me. As I reached climax, my moan of delight quickly turned to heaving bouts of anguish as I began to sob uncontrollably.

I cried for myself, for my friendship, for what I allowed Ted to do, and for what I once stopped. I cried for the little girl who went away that night on the mountain so many years ago when I was sexually assaulted. I sat up in the tub, slipped my arms around myself, and hugged myself as I rocked back and forth, crying harder than I had ever remembered. I thought about all the damage I had done to my body, all the men I had allowed to touch me and enter me. I felt sick as bursts of tears just kept spilling out of my eyes. I felt so violated and ashamed of myself and the lack of respect I enabled for so many years.

When you don't know yourself, it is so easy to allow others to define you, and that was what I did for so many years. I let friends, family, and others use me and define me and do what they wanted because I had no spine, no sense of worth.

I would assume that when most people masturbate, they just enjoy the sheer beauty and ecstasy of it all, but for me, as a rape survivor, it brought more sadness and confusion than pleasure. It turned a moan of delight into a cry of emotional pain. My sexuality was so intermingled with the bad sexual experiences I had had that it was hard for me to know and understand what a good touch is as opposed to all the bad touches over the years. Having been violated in my past, my identity and sexuality had been taken from me as well.

Learning how to love yourself and touch yourself and stay connected to all those feelings is a very hard task for any rape survivor. The violence perpetrated onto our skin has sunk in so deep that it permeates every pore, preventing us from really soaking in fully any joyful or innocent sexual experiences. The trauma resurfaces in our minds and spirits with each touch. Our skin has memory like foam, and we reshape into the curdled mass of nerves and fear we were on the night we were violated. It is why on most nights I still leave the light on, because the dark scares me.

This will be a process for me, I realized—a long process of healing and trusting and recovery, from not only drugs and alcohol, but also from self-loathing, confusion, and violation. I prayed the innocence that was stolen from me so many years ago would reemerge.

I stayed wrapped up in myself like this for a long time. It felt as though the tub drained of water and filled with my tears. Waves of emotion kept coming and crashing over me. Instead of trying to detach or stop them as I always had done in the past, I just rode them out, feeling certain they would take me under and spill over the side of the tub and drown me. But they didn't. They rose and fell in and around me like a hurricane as I screamed and cried out from this large, spinning hole that was opening up inside me, splashing emotions all over the place.

After what felt like hours, I began to calm down and pulled the drain plug from the tub. When I stood up and stepped out of the tub, I rubbed the steam off the bathroom mirror and stared at the reflection of blotchy red puffiness starring back at me. But something looked clearer. I thought I saw a little bit deeper into my blue eyes. I crawled into bed and slept more soundly than I ever remembered, awaking the next day refreshed and somehow much lighter in spirit. I was on a new journey to discover myself and had a giddy excitement in my belly about what I was going to discover.

15

Who's That Girl?

My therapist was working with me on my self-image. I truly had no idea what that was. After everything that had happened with Ted and Kathy, I started to feel good about myself. I was walking around on a little bit of a high, armed with some good, healthy experiences and decisions behind me. So in keeping with the roller coaster ride of recovery, I guess my therapist thought it was now time to dig a bit deeper and take my self-discovery to another level. It seemed like every time I made progress, I was then forced to go further down a path of wellness, which inevitably then brought back up some hurtful experience or shame or issue I had. So my mini-self-esteem rush was quickly halted when she began challenging me about the way I dressed and presented myself.

I was always a girl who was dressed up. I bought funky dresses and wore chunky high heels that resembled bowling shoes. I spent hours on my hair and makeup trying to match myself perfectly to the models in *Vogue* magazine. I was always trying on a new persona. Sometimes I braided my hair and wore shiny silver shirts with short "Catholic girl" skirts and boots; other times I wore long, flowing dresses and resembled a seventies hipster.

I was also addicted to trends and always bought the latest fashions. A slave to whatever fashion magazines said was cool that week, I had no clue what I was without the outward appearance of rebellion that most of my clothing conveyed. I was overly provocative in most of my outfits, teasing everyone with my vast cleavage or wearing T-shirts that rode up my backside, exposing a little thong or crack for the viewing pleasure of anyone behind me. I had that "hey, look at me, I'm hot shit" attitude, but then if you dared to stare too long I would snarl at you. I was a hot mess is what I was, just a very sad and lost girl.

What I really needed was love, acceptance, and someone to notice me in a nonsexual, caring, parental kind of way. But I craved the attention of others because it was the only way I knew love. The only way I could measure my self-worth was in direct proportion to the amount of attention I received on any given day, whether positive or negative attention. If I wasn't getting the attention I felt I needed, I would do things to obtain it. I might say something completely ridiculous to pull the focus onto myself or act out in an absurd manner, knowing that someone was bound to notice. I was the class clown, the first one to break the silence with some over-the-top comment bound to elicit a response. I fed off attention like a spring flower craves the rain. It raised me up and kept me high on the allure of false self-esteem and confidence. When I didn't get it, I crashed back down to the ground, falling into a vast tunnel of depression and self-loathing. It was a rapid shift from one extreme to the other and back.

My therapist and sponsor both assured me this was normal for addicts. Having never really lived life with any degree of honesty, it would be hard to actually know who I was without having many days of recovery under my belt. I just prayed they were right, because I still felt so fucking uncomfortable in my skin that I wanted to crawl out of it.

It had been easier before to hide beneath the high, to create the self I thought the world wanted and remain high enough to not really care that I was all fake nails and hair dye. I didn't know who the girl in the mirror was, and I had no idea what this body was supposed to do and how I should have felt or even what I should have worn. I always dressed up like a Barbie doll, emulating what I saw in magazines, on TV, and in the shadows of my mind—I didn't know what *I* really wanted.

I didn't leave the house without makeup because I hated my skin underneath. I hated the vulnerability my face exposed without heavy black eyeliner and bright, fully lined lips. I wore different-colored contacts all the time to change my view, and I colored my hair more frequently than the seasons changed the leaves from green to red. I changed everything. I transformed the outside to figure out whether it matched the inside. Nothing made me feel complete, just covered up enough to blend in.

Dressing provocatively, or "in character," had worked for me while I was using, but now being in recovery, I was lost in this state of total confusion as to who I was and what that should look like. One thing was certain: I was no longer "that" girl, and now with the gentle prodding of my therapist, we would have to piece together who this new girl was and what she should look like.

16

PSEUDO-LESBIAN

I BEGAN TAKING AN INTEREST IN AN OLDER LESBIAN IN my meetings. A small clique of them sat together at meetings and I started to gravitate toward them. I felt a connection that I couldn't place. I became friends with them and began going to dinner with them after meetings and hanging out with them on the weekends.

I was slowly becoming part of their crew, even though I was not yet identifying myself as a lesbian. I knew I considered myself bisexual based on my past experiences, and that was about as far as I was willing to go in the acceptance department at that point. My sponsor Rose was a part of this group, so hanging around her provided me with a great excuse to latch onto them all. I still had all kinds of confusion and fear built up inside me about my sexuality. But I knew I felt safe with these women, and I felt a kinship with them that was so nice that I just went along with it. They never questioned me or my intent; they just accepted me as one of their own.

One woman in particular, Lynn, caught my eye, and she and I became great friends. I loved hanging out with her. We started calling each other on the phone incessantly and would talk for hours. There was an ease in the conversation that was wonderfully simple. I didn't have to search my brain for topics or conversation starters; thoughts just flowed from our mouths like water and seemed to endlessly stream on and on. Eventually she became the first call I made in the morning and the last call I made at night. She always gave me that little belly-flipping feeling when I would encounter her with her short, graying brown, butch-cut hair and masculine facial features.

She looked visibly weathered, and her hands were rough and clearly had been used plenty. I was drawn to her in an odd way—not so much in a physical or sexual way, but in an "I would love to be your best friend," intriguing way.

I have had crushes on females since kindergarten, and although I attempted to pretend these feelings didn't exist, I always knew deep down that they never went away. In my drug-using past, I'd had random hook-ups with a couple of women, but I always discounted them, saying, "I was drunk" or "I was just experimenting," and I went about my heterosexual lifestyle. All the while, the thoughts and feelings lingered inside me. In recovery, as I began to be honest with myself and take this journey of self-discovery, I was finding myself once again drawn to women.

I had thought a lot about what my therapist and I had talked about regarding the way I dressed and how I carried myself. I began to explore different ideas of clothing and my self-image. My new friends were very different from the people I had hung out with in my past. They were casual and not slaves to trends, as I had always tried to be. They would often comment on my midriff shirt or my pants that were so low my underwear was showing. They confronted me in gentle ways, asking if I was trying to get attention. They asked me whether I really wanted all eyes on me. I started to take cues from them and began transforming my wardrobe. Lynn and I went shopping at stores I never would have shopped in before because I saw their clothes as nerdy or conservative.

Gradually, I began trading my halter tops and low riders for polo shirts and cargo pants. As I got comfortable with this clothing transformation, I realized it felt good to be covered up and not have men staring at me like the piece of meat they thought I was and that I had placed out before them so eagerly. Under this new layer of clothes, I was safe to try to explore who the person was inside.

As the days, nights, and weekends that Lynn and I spent together began to string on and on, I found myself in a pseudo-lesbian relationship. I say pseudo because the most intimacy that ever resulted was long and inappropriate hugging and snuggling. I was enjoying her company and learning how to be intimate emotionally with another person, which was something I had yet to really accomplish. We would sit around and talk about everything, and we began to share this wonderful bond that felt safe and secure. The fact that there was no sexual intimacy was a plus for me. I was still very confused about my sexuality and needed a nice, long break in the activity in that department. We slept together almost every night but nothing ever happened. It was nice to have a relationship (with sex nowhere in the picture) that felt so much more intimate than any of my past relationships. Sex used to be the glue that held together the farce of intimacy for me. I felt great comfort in just being with someone without the demand of my body as the ultimate price.

Lynn also told me about the depths of her pain and her past experiences, some that mirrored mine and others that were just horrific. While the strands of this extremely intimate dialogue slowly wove themselves into a comfortable and warm relationship, I found myself opening up to her in ways I had never done with anyone before, telling her things that I had only mentioned in my journal. Sharing my deepest fears and doubts with her felt so natural. When she questioned me about my past, I didn't become defensive or shut down like I usually did with people. Instead, I allowed myself to feel, to trust, and to share my most private thoughts with her.

I had always been reluctant to trust anyone, thinking that the person probably had ulterior motives. But Lynn was gentle with me, and kind. She wanted nothing more from me than I was willing to give on any given day.

For once, someone was interested in my thoughts, ideas, and, most importantly, my feelings. She held them all in the palm of her hand in such a gentle manner that I didn't know how to begin to dissect it all, so instead I just fell into the relationship and relished this new feeling of intimacy that was so foreign to me.

17

MOURNING

ONE NIGHT DURING ONE OF THE THOUSANDS OF DEEP
conversations Lynn and I had, the subject of my mother's death came
up, a topic I had rarely spoken about since getting into recovery. At the
very mention of it, I started to cry. I started and didn't stop. Suddenly
this floodgate in me opened up, and I began to dump my emotions all
over her lap. I cried and cried, harder and heavier than I had ever done
in the presence of another person—heaving sobs that I usually reserved
for the privacy of my bathtub. I found myself hyperventilating and
snotting all over my pseudo-lesbian girlfriend. She just held me and
comforted me. She wiped my tears away and brushed my hair away
from my wet face, just as I had always envisioned people doing for
others they loved. I felt incredibly secure in her arms. For the first time,
I felt I could be truly and uncharacteristically vulnerable with another
human, free from the usual fears that stopped my tears from flowing
and forced my body upright into a protective manner I would retreat

to when things got too deep for me to handle. On this night, I just allowed myself to crumple into her chest and let the feelings seep out of me.

I fell asleep crying that night. When I woke up, I was still sobbing. My pillow was so wet that it was evident I had been crying all night in my sleep. Lynn had to go to work, so I was left alone. I called off work at the travel agency because even as I made the phone call, I could barely speak; I was heaving so hard with emotion. When lunchtime came and went and there seemed no end to my tears, I called my therapist's office, sure that I was having a breakdown of some sort, since I had already gone through two boxes of tissues. I was thankful that she was able to fit me into her afternoon appointments. I attempted to take a shower but ended up falling against the wall in sobs. This was ridiculous, I thought. I couldn't stop no matter how hard I tried. The tears kept coming like a harsh spring rain on a windowsill. They spilled down my face with no end in sight.

As I sat in my therapist's office, crying all over myself and clinging to multiple wadded-up tissues, I looked at her and shook my head back and forth. "I don't know what is wrong with me," I said, and went on to explain that the previous night I had just been talking about my mother's death, and suddenly—waterworks! As I continued to ramble about not understanding what was happening, my therapist gently leaned toward me and put her hand on my knee. "Jennifer, what you're experiencing is very normal and, well, very long overdue," she said. "You are grieving for the loss of your mother—finally!" I just looked at her with a blank face. Well, that explanation had never dawned on me.

I thought I had already grieved for her loss. After all, I had cried in the hospital and at the funeral. During the weeks leading up to her death, I had somehow managed to not drink. I had been on autopilot, walking around like a robot doing everything I needed to do for her, but that was all; I was doing, but not feeling. Back then, I deployed my standard detachment defensive mechanisms to get through it all.

Then, immediately after her funeral, I walked directly into a bar, took my seat upon my escape perch, and basically didn't leave that stool for three months. That binge eventually culminated in my suicide attempt, which landed me in rehab, and eventually led me to this much softer seat in my therapist's office. She went on to explain that I had never really dealt with my pain appropriately. I may have cried at all the right times and places, but then I went on to get high for three months.

I began to protest, to tell her that I had spoken about it often, that in the halfway house I had even bought a balloon for my mother, written a letter to her, tied it to the balloon, and released it, thinking for certain that all of my emotions must have traveled away with the balloon as it launched itself into the sky. I went on to tell her of my annoying habit when I got high with friends of telling them my whole life story. Almost robotically, I would take them through the most horrifying, intimate details of my sexual abuse history, my mother's death, everything. And I kept a straight face and felt strong when I did it. It was as if I was saying, "Look what I went though. See how easily I can talk about these horrible events and they don't even bother me? I am a soldier. Can't you see my strength?" I could recite my own pain with no emotion. In some twisted way, I thought I was healing and that talking about it in this way was good for me. But as my therapist explained, without the emotion to accompany the words, it was as though I was saying nothing at all.

Emotional detachment was a not-so-good tool I had carried into recovery with me. I was the queen of emotional detachment. It was a survival skill I had developed and could perform on cue if need be. I talked a lot at meetings and in therapy about my past but still hadn't reached the point where I actually *felt* my past. This was most likely because I never allowed myself to feel anything. When feelings came up for me in the past, I drank or used to cover them. I never indulged them, or even labeled them for that matter. In rehab and in the halfway house, I had some good breakthroughs, as they call them in therapy, surrounding my past sexual assaults, but had yet to fully grasp the concept of this new way of dealing with things. I had to learn how to pair my emotions with my experiences and do so appropriately. This was all so new to me and so incredibly hard. I could look you in the face, deadpan, and tell you everything about myself with vivid details, but to allow myself the vulnerability of showing you my feelings that stirred underneath—that was another story.

And yet, here I was, crying freely in front of two people on two different days. This was serious progress.

I left my therapist's office wondering when I would stop crying. She had said that I could go through this for a couple of days, that I was experiencing a long-overdue mourning period for my mother and I needed to just settle into my grief and deal with it. So I decided to indulge my newfound sorrow and went to the store and bought more tissues and a pint of ice cream—mind you, I was still crying the whole time I selected the items and made my purchase. By this time my eyes were beyond red, puffy and swollen, and people were looking at me funny, but I didn't care. I walked through the grocery store with a new badge of entitlement. I felt oddly strong in my sudden comfort with outward emotion, as though it were some shiny armor I had discovered.

At home, I popped my copy of *Beaches* into the video player. I figured if I was going to be in this state, I might as well crank it up a notch and watch the most gut-wrenchingly heartbreaking movie of all time. Besides, I had first watched it with my mother, and it always reminded me of her. I cried even harder while watching the movie.

Then I called my employer and said I needed to take a couple of bereavement days off to mourn the loss of my mother. My boss immediately was sympathetic as she told me it was okay and to take all the time I needed. I thanked her profusely, and then she asked how and when it happened. When I told her it was almost two years ago, there was dead silence on the phone. Still sobbing, I tried to explain that I hadn't dealt with it before, and I was now finally processing all my feelings. My boss's sympathy dried up and her tone grew angry as she began to recite the agency's policy on bereavement and informed me that my current situation didn't really fall within that policy. I explained that there was no way I could come in under my current circumstance and that I had no idea when I would be suitable for public consumption. Needless to say, I was fired. Great, I thought— just more reason to add to my already overflowing waterworks.

So I settled in and spent the next three days mourning as I pored over pictures of my mother and me together, watched a video I had of us at Christmastime, and read over cards she had sent. I had saved almost every one from my sweet sixteenth birthday until the last card she sent me just months before her death. I avoided the phone when it rang, and I simply self-indulged. I didn't shower or change my clothes. I just sat and cried and ate ice cream and watched sad movies and listened to Sarah McLachlan CDs. Surely it was a combination for a complete and utter emotional breakdown, and I was game. It was about time. My framework had stood tall and sturdy for too many years, taking in all the horrible shit I and others had put me through without ever wavering. Now it was all crashing down around me, and I was dancing among the ruins.

I emerged from my apartment three days later, refreshed and with a peaceful calm that was unbelievable. I had thoroughly processed through my pain and emotions and felt lighter than I had ever felt before. This recovery emotional-cleansing stuff was tough, but the feeling of freedom that followed was incredible.

18

ANNIVERSARY

SOME IN RECOVERY BELIEVE THAT IF YOU ARE NOT
in pain, then you are not changing or growing. You have to physically
and emotionally walk through your pain to get to the other side of
it. While I was using this was never an option for me, because the
emotional mountains I had created in my life seemed far too high to
climb. Now in recovery, even though I cannot see the beautiful clearing
on the other side of the mountain, I know it is there, so I just have to
push myself up that emotional and at times very painful and steep path
to get to the other side—one step at a time. As clichéd as that sounds,
it is so true.

After coming out of mourning for my mother, I had no idea
what the next step would be for me, especially since I no longer
had a job, but I put one foot in front of the other and it was slowly
revealed. I spent that fall continuing to do the next right thing, going

to meetings, sharing my feelings with others, talking to my therapist, and just plain enjoying the new energy I had for life. My parents were taking care of my bills with some of the money I still had left from my mother's settlement, so I didn't have to get a job right away. I felt as though anything was possible and that the world was at my fingertips. Truthfully, I had no idea what I wanted to do or become, but simply the thought that I could do anything was empowering and thrilling.

I was coming up on the elusive one-year anniversary in the program, and I had a lot of anticipation about reaching it. In recovery, we count time because it is a valid and validating way to chart your growth. Everyone always knows exactly how much time in recovery they have—in fact, if you ask, some recovering people can even tell you to the minute. The year was a landmark. It was a full twelve months, fifty-two weeks, 365 days, 8,760 hours, or 525,600 minutes without picking up a drink or drug. It's a birthday in many ways, and it becomes just as important, if not more important, than your actual birthday. For so many of us, it is when our lives truly begin to take form and productive shape, as opposed to all the useless drunken months, days, and hours we had spent withering away before. It is an accomplishment not to be overlooked but to be celebrated. In many meetings, the year is an indescribable goal that many try to achieve but few actually do. Recovery is hard, and the first year is often the hardest. So many people relapse within the first year that many meetings even have rules about it, for example:

- You shouldn't date in the first year.

- You cannot share your story until you have a full year of recovery.

- You cannot lead a meeting until you have a full year of recovery.

- You shouldn't sponsor anyone else in the first year.

The rules contributed to making the first-year anniversary an incredible goal to reach, one that brought with it a level of respect from others in meetings.

On or immediately after the one-year anniversary, meeting leaders suggest and sometimes request that a person share his or her story in a speaker meeting. It is recommended that the speaker share for the entirety of the meeting, which is usually an hour. This is a great rite of passage in many recovery places, and I was eager for my turn. I had been counting down my months, weeks, and days like a small child counting down to Christmas or the start of summer.

The ritual of handing out the chips is an important part of the meeting. It is always done either at the beginning or the end of the meeting. Various lengths of recovery are called out, and one by one people walk up to the front of the room and claim their prized chip denoting the length of time in recovery. I collected all my colorful, plastic round chips along the way—twenty-four hours, thirty days, sixty days, and ninety days. As people receive their chips, the group always applauds and hoots and hollers, and a lot of hugging occurs.

But the one-year chip—oh, that was a different thing altogether. First of all, it wasn't plastic; it was a medallion of sorts. It wasn't colorful; it was a solid bronze metal coin twice the thickness of other chips to represent the newfound stability in life after having achieved a year. Many meeting-goers have a saying when handing them out: "Put this in your mouth, and if it melts, then you can drink." The round of applause is usually the loudest when people get their first one-year chip. As someone who often had dramatic scenes playing in my head with me as the star, I envisioned myself going up to the front of the room and graciously accepting my one-year medallion with all the humility of a starlet winning an Oscar. In my daydream, I dramatically thanked my sponsor and the rooms of recovery, instead of the Academy, before chanting, "You like me; you really like me."

This would be a really big deal for me.

I was asked to tell my story at a Friday night meeting, which was always one of the larger meetings in town. I was giddy, nervous, and excited. I had never spoken for a whole hour in front of a group of people before. During the past few months, I had been sharing for three to five minutes at some meetings, and even then I always got sweaty palms and a shaky voice. It scared the crap out of me to open up my mouth and speak my truth in a room full of strangers. But that is what recovery is all about—sharing our experience, strength, and hope with others so that they may understand what the program is like and how it works. In essence, this is why twelve-step recovery works. Without the meetings and other addicts sharing their stories with one another, it would be much harder for people to understand how to make it one day at a time. We lean on each other; it is a *we* program, not an *I* program.

Even though I had sat through hours and hours of meetings, I can honestly say that I took something positive away from every meeting I attended. I may not have always liked the messenger, but as my sponsor Rose always said, "Principles over personalities." She repeated this slogan to me often—so much that I felt as though it should be tattooed to my forehead. I didn't always like everyone in the rooms. There were all types of people at meetings, and I had a tendency to be a little judgmental. Every time I started talking shit about someone, there would be Rose saying, "Jennifer, principles over personalities. Hear the message and ignore the messenger." And believe it or not, when I opened my mind up enough to actually listen, I learned the most from those I disliked the most.

Rose was a great sponsor and really guided me through those months. I called her daily, chatting away about the events of my day, my frustrations, fears, successes, joys, and everything in between. She was always there to listen and offer strong, recovery-oriented advice. Being new in the program, I didn't have the best patience. After all, most addicts have a slogan of their own: "I want what I want and I want it *now*!" When I was having one of my moments of utter frustration over something, her classic response to me was always "This too shall pass." I grew to hate that phrase, not because it wasn't true—it was the absolute truth—but because I was so impatient so often that Rose said it to me daily, sometimes multiple times a day. It got to the point where every time she said it to me, I would mimic it back to her in a childlike tone and then add, "like whole corn through my ass." She always laughed off my defiance because she knew I was only joking, which I was. Rose had such a great sense of humor, and we laughed a lot. She had a gentle way of guiding me into the right frame of mind. Her sense of humor was so much like those of people I had grown up with that she instantly felt familial, and that worked for me. She gave me a daily devotional book that ended up becoming my saving grace at times when I needed it most. Each morning, I opened this book and it always managed to have the exact message or lesson that I needed that day.

At my one-year anniversary, she also gave me another gift that I loved and wore daily. It was a little gold charm that held the Serenity Prayer gently carved into its thin, flat frame. It was a charm that all the women in our group received when they had a year of recovery. It was a sign of passage, if you will, among this amazing group of women who all cared for and loved each other so much. We were one another's strength in times of great weakness. I placed it on a long, gold chain that my mother used to wear and that I inherited after she passed away. The charm fell slightly above my heart, which was exactly where I needed it to be at all times.

My parents decided to make the trip to State College to hear me give my lead, which is another way of saying my sharing of my story for the first time. I was so incredibly nervous that I thought I might puke. In fact, as I sat there on a wooden stool in front of about fifty people, including my sponsor and parents, I started off my lead by saying, "I think I might puke," which got a laugh out of everyone and put me at ease a bit. My palms were sweaty as I started from the beginning and talked about the reasons I used, the things that happened to me as a result of my using, the people I hurt, the things I lost, the trouble I got into, how I almost died, how I eventually got into recovery, and how incredibly different my life was today.

It wasn't until I sat there and told my story that I realized how far I had come. What a miracle I was! How amazing this program was!

By the end of my story I was beaming with pride, and yet had humility so raw that I cried openly. The audience burst into applause, and I was enthralled with the response. Seeing the utter pride on my parents' faces was indescribable. Their eyes glowed as they beamed at me. It was such an unfamiliar response—I had been so accustomed to placing pain directly into those patient and loving eyes and seeing it staring back at me. So this pride, this joyful look in their eyes broke my heart, but in a good way.

As my parents and others began to swarm around me and hug me, I can honestly say that I had never felt unconditional love and joy like that before. It was overwhelming. In addition to my dad and my stepmom, my sponsor and my friends in recovery had become my new family. I felt so blessed. Just when I thought things couldn't get any better in recovery, I turned a corner or reached a milestone and things got better. I was beginning to live this life that had been beyond my wildest expectations.

MORE WILL BE REVEALED

I used the Serenity Prayer

in every aspect of my life

and believed strongly in the part that says

"the courage to change the things I can."

19

APPLYING MYSELF

I'D MADE IT TO MY ONE-YEAR RECOVERY ANNIVERSARY, but I still faced many challenges. I hadn't found a job and my money was running out, so I had to make some sort of decision regarding my future. My therapist introduced the idea of college to me during one of our sessions. I had begun to think that going to school might be a good next step for me, although I wasn't sure I would be able to go because of finances and my past horrible grades. My former grade point average was a 1.5; a scholarly asset I was not.

My therapist introduced me to a guy from the Office of Rehabilitation Vocation. He told me that I could apply to Pennsylvania State University as a provisional student, which basically meant they would accept me as a student, but I would be placed on probation for the first year. I filled out the application and wrote an essay explaining why I wanted to attend college. I wrote about my past drinking and drug use and about why my grades were so bad. I wrote about my mom and how losing her was my breaking point. I finished the essay by telling them how I went to a rehabilitation program, then moved to State College to start a new life, and that I had been in recovery for more than a year.

In many ways, I gave Penn State an abbreviated version of my fourth step. A fourth step in recovery is a moral inventory of your past, or, in other words, a written depiction of all the things you did in your addiction that you need to make amends for—whether those amends are with yourself, your higher power, or other people in your life. It is usually done within the first year, but it can vary depending upon a person's willingness and emotional and spiritual growth. Many people dread this step and avoid it like the plague. It requires you to take a painstakingly hard look at yourself and your actions. Being the big old nerd that I had become in early recovery, I didn't shy away from this task at all; in fact, I was excited about it. One of the things that really clicked with me early on when I was in the rehabilitation center was that I had to revisit everything in my past and dig up all my issues and deal with them if I didn't want to relapse. The fourth step to me was to be a huge scooping out of myself all the crap I had allowed drugs and alcohol to do to me. I sat down one night and began typing. I used a recovery book to help guide me in format, and just began to write. It was then that I fell back in love with the art of writing and realized how much I had missed it. I used to write all the time as a young person— poems, short stories, etc. I actually still have the first short story I ever wrote when I was fifteen (I got an A!). By the time I was done I had typed over ten pages, single-spaced. It was emotionally exhausting, and I learned more about my past than I thought I knew. It was another cleansing. When most people think of a moral inventory, they think of some dark and scary task, but it actually left me feeling light and free, as though a huge burden had been lifted from me.

After having done a fourth step, the college essay was easy for me. I mailed the essay and application with no expectations at all. I didn't fear judgment, because I knew that today my life was good and my past mistakes only made me stronger. I didn't obsess about whether or not I would get in; I just kind of sent it off into the universe. If it's meant to be, then it's meant to be, I thought. This was another gift of recovery that was so strong in my life by this time. I just knew things would be okay. I knew I wouldn't always get what I wanted, but somehow I would always get what I needed.

Lo and behold, several months later, a letter arrived in my mailbox. As I tore through it, I saw the wording: "Congratulations, you have been accepted...." I almost fainted! Never in a million years would I have guessed that I would be going to college. The pride that began to swell up in my heart was overwhelming. I did it. I was worth something. At least to Penn State University, I was someone; I was a student.

I immediately called my parents to tell them the good news, and they shared in my delight. I could hear the pride and joy in their voices as they told me how proud they were of me and that it was so exciting. I hung up the phone in amazement. My life had done such a turnabout. These types of conversations were becoming the norm with my parents, and that in and of itself was odd. I usually disappointed them and made excuses for my behavior. But lately it was the other way around, and I began to feel proud of myself and excited to share my daily activities and achievements with them.

I started to feel valid, as though I actually might have a purpose after all. No one in my family had ever come close to going to college, let alone gotten into a major top-ten university. A new chapter in my life was about to begin; I was to start college in mid-January, and I couldn't even put into words the thrill I felt.

Yet I had all the fears of any person starting something for the first time. Could I handle classes, tests, and homework? Had I fried too many brain cells to excel? To deal with the fears, I shared my concerns in my meetings. The great thing about people in recovery is their unconditionally supportive nature. I was able to place my fears at the feet of my peers, and they picked them up and held them for me. They reassured me that I would make it and that I deserved to be in college. I still was battling internal self-worth issues, which are so common in early recovery. People in recovery believed in me, sometimes before I believed in me. I had become good at verbalizing my fears when I needed to, before they festered inside me and became issues. I had been working so hard at getting myself emotionally healthy, and I felt ready to take on a new challenge.

20

MIXED MESSAGES

I WAS SLOWLY FORMING A WONDERFUL NEW BOND
with my parents. They were becoming so important in my life. My
relationship with them before recovery was built on falsehoods and
manipulations. I was always trying to hide my true self from them,
and they were always pretending not to really see me. We did this
uncomfortable dance around each other that never allowed us to get to
truly know each other. By avoiding the land mines around us that none
of us wanted to talk about, we avoided any form of intimacy other
than the rare glimpses when I invited, or should I say *pulled* them into
the hole I was living in by sheer desperation. Like when I got pregnant
at nineteen and needed to tell them. They helped me make a tough
decision, and my father walked me through my abortion. Or when I
tried to kill myself, and it was their answering machine that blinked
with the horrible news of my nearly successful suicide attempt in 1997.

Now that it was 1999 and I was in recovery, almost all my skeletons were out of the closet and there wasn't much my parents didn't know about me and my past—except for one thing. Sometimes I would borrow my pseudo-girlfriend's nice new SUV and drive it home on the weekends to see my parents, and they would question me as to whose car it was. I would just say it was a friend's car and blow it off. I wasn't quite ready to tell them that I was in an emotionally safe, nonsexual, pseudo-lesbian relationship. It was best that they just believed I was happy and working on myself and making new friends in State College. I am sure they noticed the rainbow on the back of the car, or the fact that many of the friends who were at my one-year lecture were oddly butch; but if they did, they didn't say a word.

As Christmas approached, I went out shopping and bought all types of little gifts for Lynn and a beautiful, sappy-as-hell card that expressed my undying love for her. It was a little over the top, but I was just thrilled to have someone to spend the holiday with and wanted it to be really special. I allowed myself to get all wrapped up in the holiday spirit and what it means when you're in a relationship. I did the same for everyone in my family; I wanted to give cards that really expressed how much I loved everyone, and I took special care picking out each card. Lynn and I decided we would exchange our gifts upon my arrival home from spending Christmas with my parents.

I went home and had a wonderful Christmas with my parents and saw my brothers and niece. My brothers were still looking rough; they had been partying hard and it was still all the same drama with them. But like always in our family, no one ever misses a Christmas holiday. Christmas in our house was a monumental event, and we were always overly spoiled. We all opened our cards and presents and it was wonderful in those moments. I only stayed for three days, and that was just enough to get my dose of home and the drama that came with it all. I drove back to State College in excited anticipation of my first Christmas with Lynn. As we sat in my apartment with our individual piles of gifts ready for presentation, we handed each other a card to start. I read the one she gave me, and it was a beautiful, flower-filled love note as worthy as the one I'd picked out for her; but when I lifted my tear-filled eyes to look at her, I was immediately struck by the contorted, confused look on her face.

She just looked up at me and said, "Umm, I know I am older than you, but this card says, 'To My Loving Parents.'" My heart dropped and my eyes widened. "*What!*" I yelped, ripping the card from her hand. Sure enough, it read, "To My Loving Parents" on the front. As the realization of what had happened sunk in a little deeper, my heart was now occupying a space in the bottom of my shoe. I must have mixed up the cards as I was stuffing them into their respective envelopes. I quickly picked up her envelope, and sure enough, her name was on the front in my handwriting, but the card was for my parents, which meant the card my parents opened... "Oh my god," I stuttered over and over again. She tried calming me down, but I was in full-blown panic mode by that point and trying to replay every second of my visit home. Surely my parents would have said something if they saw that their Christmas card was really a mushy love card written out to another woman, wouldn't they?

I was totally freaking out, and Lynn's attempts to try and calm me down weren't working at all. A ton of questions were flying around in my head and coming out of my mouth in rapid fashion as I paced the floor of my living room: "They would have said something, right?" "They must not have really read the card." "Maybe they were just being nice and didn't know what to say." "Oh my god, what if they think I am gay?" I was hyperventilating, and needless to say, the mood was killed and we spent the rest of the night analyzing every potential scenario that could have happened and might yet happen. I could tell Lynn was slightly put off by my reaction of utter disgust and fear that my parents might find out about her. Even though she understood the issues of coming out to parents and the realities that major decision held for most people, I could still tell she was hurt and took it personally. I felt terrible about it and tried to explain to her that it wasn't about her, it was just that I still had no idea what I was doing and who I was, so there was no way I was ready to try and explain it to my parents.

Over the next days, I called home frequently, checking in, making small talk, and mentioning how nice this Christmas was with all the cards, presents, etc. They never said anything or let on for a second that anything was off. After a week or two with no confrontation from them and no indication whatsoever that they knew, I began to breathe a sigh of relief. Maybe they just didn't read it that closely, which then kind of pissed me off since I had taken amazing care picking out the card, and then they never read it.

I talked about it in my weekly therapy sessions and began to look at my sexuality a bit deeper. I was trying to figure out exactly what I was doing with Lynn. Again, my therapist was gentle and nonjudgmental and let me talk freely about my confusion without having to come to any concrete solutions. She said that sexuality is sometimes fluid and what I was exploring was totally normal and okay. It was so nice to have someone so incredibly unconditional to talk to.

21

Smoke Screens

New Year's Eve was quickly approaching, and I
decided it was time to end my one lingering, nasty addiction: smoking.
I had smoked cigarettes since I was eleven years old. Day in and day
out, those little tobacco-filled tubes were a part of my life. Never
in a million years would I have thought that I would give them up.
However, recently I had noticed that I was getting out of breath just
from climbing a small flight of steps. I was also becoming more aware
of the stench of smoke, and I didn't like what I smelled. I had said
early on in my recovery that I would wait at least a year before I would
consider quitting smoking. I knew trying to quit everything at once
would have been way too hard, so I kept the habit as long as I could.

My life was becoming so clean and so pure that the whole smoking
thing just didn't fit me anymore. The cigarettes looked odd in my hand
as I carried them around. They no longer matched the person smoking

them, and I began to feel slightly hypocritical each time I would light one up. Here I was with over a year in recovery, trying to live a life of brutal honesty and integrity, yet I was still addicted to a drug that I used every hour, if not more. It didn't feel right to me anymore, and I wasn't enjoying them like I used to. I wanted to be totally healthy, and smoking no longer fit into the new lifestyle I was living.

I started smoking like a chimney—not that I wasn't smoking that way to begin with, since I smoked about two packs a day—but in preparation for quitting. I forced myself to literally chain-smoke for the week leading up to my final day. I had heard of people doing this before quitting to make themselves just sick to death of smoking. So I fired up one nasty butt after another while sitting in my living room watching TV. As soon as I would crush one out into the ashtray, I would immediately light up another one. My ashtray was overflowing, and after a day or two of this, I swear my face was turning a gross shade of green. On New Year's Eve, Lynn and I went to a party with a bunch of recovering people and played games all night. Lynn was a heavy smoker too and decided that she would quit with me. We made our pact that just before midnight, we would smoke one last cigarette and then flush the rest down the toilet. I was determined not to smoke again. Now that I had made the decision, that was it; my mind was made up! Lynn wasn't as committed, and I think she was doing it more for me than for herself. I knew that once I quit I would never be able to date a smoker again—I just knew the smell and taste would make me want to throw up. I knew Lynn would have a harder time doing this, which could have been my subconscious way to sabotage the relationship. But for now, we were doing this together.

So at midnight, we both sucked away on our last cigarette. I pulled hard off my former best friend and inhaled deeper than I ever had until the red cherry burned all the way down to my fingers and all that was left was a brown filter. "That's it," I said as I dumped my pack of cigarettes into the toilet. Watching the loose tobacco freeing itself and rising up in the water like tea from a bag that had just burst open in a cup of water, I realized my love affair with smoking was coming to an abrupt halt. I reached for the lever to flush the toilet with a tinge of sadness. These were my first vices, my first drug, and my first rite of passage into the destructive path I ended up stumbling down for years. Cigarettes were always there, no matter what, through thick and thin. I could light up a cigarette just about anywhere and get at least a hint of a high when I needed it. You don't realize how much you smoke until, well, until you don't. Smoking is the most socially acceptable form of drug abuse in the country, and up until recent years, you could smoke everywhere. It was universally accepted and embraced, making it one of the deadliest and most cunning manifestations of addiction to try to break away from.

But I was determined, and as I was beginning to learn in my recovery, my determination was actually quite fierce. Once I set my sights on something, I went after it with every fiber of my being. This newfound sense of empowerment and accomplishment was strange to me but quickly became one of my favorite things about recovery. I could do things. I could dream. I could achieve. I followed through. These were all things I never believed in my addiction. I couldn't or wouldn't have even tried to follow through with anything that seemed worthwhile because I never believed in myself enough to give anything a fighting chance. It was just easier to be self-defeating about things than to challenge myself and risk failure. So, after having a over a year of recovery under my belt and a letter from Pennsylvania State University that said I was worthy enough to at least be on probation with them and become a student, I was ready to tackle anything.

It was hard—harder than I ever in a million years would have imagined. It wasn't the kind of craving that went away. It was as though someone had pushed the fast-forward button on my thoughts. Everything was flying around in my head at a speed that was physically exhausting. I had an energy surge that ripped through my body and made me physically shake from its impact on my skin for days. I was vibrating. I was a maniac. This is apparently a common side effect of quitting smoking. I had no idea and was totally unprepared for this reaction. I hadn't had any major physical withdrawal symptoms from alcohol and drugs.

My thoughts ran across my brain so fast that my mouth felt like a court reporter trying to keep up with an overly articulate judge. I would stumble over my words as I tried to speak to people or in meetings. It was embarrassing. I couldn't get the words out fast enough, and just as I would say one thought, another one ripped by like on an accelerated marquee.

I decided it was best to stay home as much as possible, but when I tried to just sit and watch TV, the vibrating started and I would get up and start cleaning or organizing. I can say this with 100 percent certainty: Quitting smoking had a highly positive effect on my apartment. I cleaned every inch of it. It had never been so squeaky-clean! On the fourth day, I decided to cleanse my whole apartment of the damage I had done by smoking. I had all this energy so I figured I might as well put it to some good use. I began with general tasks like vacuuming and dusting.

While I was scrubbing the kitchen counter with some bleach cleanser, I made the mistake of scrubbing a little mark on the wall. I was living in a standard apartment, so all of my walls had been painted white. So when I scrubbed this little section of the wall, it revealed a bright white patch of paint that apparently was suffocating underneath the layers of toxic, yellow smoke stains that had clung to my walls from my heavy smoking. I just stared at the little patch of whiteness blaring back at me from the nasty wall. It made me sick. I thought of what my lungs must look like and began scrubbing harder and harder. Before I knew it I was plowing all my manic energy into these walls, and I was on a mission to get them back to the bright white they once were. I scrubbed and scrubbed for hours until every inch of my apartment's walls was cleansed, and once I finished the last of the walls, I collapsed onto my couch and took in my work. My apartment sparkled like they do in those great Lysol commercials. It smelled sanitized, not dingy. I was finally physically exhausted, the vibrating stopped, and I was able to just breathe in a deep and cleansing breath. It felt amazing.

Lynn wasn't doing as well as I was, and she quickly lit up a cigarette after a couple days of not being able to stand not smoking. I told her she couldn't smoke in front of me or in my house. There was something about having cleansed my home and my body that made me feel refreshed, energized, and ready for change. She was bitter, angry, and beginning to become a real drain on my energy to be around.

With that in mind, I decided it was time to end my pseudo-lesbian relationship, which went over like a lead balloon with my suitor. I sat her down one day and just told her I wasn't ready for a relationship, that I was too new to recovery and going to college—I essentially made every excuse I could without saying, "I am just not into you in that way." I just knew I wasn't ready, and I wanted to walk into this college thing on my own without any ties or distractions. My whole life was in front of me, and I was eager to tackle it by myself. I tried to tell her I still wanted to be her friend, which really was what we were anyway— there was no physical intimacy, no long kissing sessions or any gestures that remotely resembled a relationship other than being inseparable all the time. But she felt for me in a way that I wasn't capable of feeling for her. She was angry and upset and wouldn't speak to me. She told me she couldn't be my friend and began to get very mean with me when we spoke.

I thought Lynn and I could transition into being friends smoothly, but boy, was I wrong. She wouldn't return my calls or even look at me in meetings other than sending a random snarl in my direction. Thus, my introduction to lesbian drama began. This, as I would come to understand, is highly common in tight-knit lesbian communities. Those who are best friends and partners one minute will break up and hate each other the next, and many times will break up and switch partners in a heartbeat, causing even more public emotional outbursts and childish antics. Yet the little circle still must find a way to function, so dramatic entertainment just becomes standard until it all blows over and the exes become best friends again and start to vacation in Provincetown, Massachusetts, during the summer with their new partners and dogs. It's complicated, as only women who love women can be. It's emotional, it's deep, it's sometimes political, and it is always personal. In lesbian relationships, rarely is *anything* left unsaid or undone.

Lynn ran around to every one of our mutual friends like a wounded cat, crying the blues to anyone who would listen and putting all of our friends and community into an uncomfortable situation. Suddenly a group of tight-knit gals was being fractured as she demanded that I not be present at events or dinners. Ironically, just as Penn State was recognizing me as accepted, I was losing acceptance among my lesbian friends.

22

STARTING SCHOOL

I DECIDED TO TAKE A STEP BACK FROM MY RECOVERY group of lesbian friends and the drama and put all my focus on my new endeavor—being a freshman at Pennsylvania State University. I felt as giddy and nerdy as I did the first day of kindergarten, when I got all dolled up in a red-and-black plaid dress with my black patent leather mary janes, hair placed tightly in pigtails on either side of my eager-to-be-educated head.

My brother Brian, who is a year and a half older than me, got to experience kindergarten a year before me, and for my overachieving self, that was unacceptable. So in my little four-year-old brain, I plotted a way to join him.

I loved spending my endless days playing with Brian. He and I were glued at the hip, and many people thought we were twins because we shared such a similar face—both blue-eyed with brown hair and a sprinkle of freckles across the bridge of the nose. We used to make up characters and tape ourselves on our little tape recorder. Two of our many characters were an old couple named George and Marcy. We would talk for hours into the tape recorder, making our voices sound like an old couple and falling into fits of giggles as we got a kick out of each other's imitations. Still to this day when I call Brian at work, I tell his coworkers that Marcy is on the phone, and he knows immediately that it is me and picks up in his "old" voice. We were inseparable, and the thought of him leaving me on a daily basis and me being alone with my mother was unbearable.

So I decided I was going to go with him to kindergarten, although I never shared this idea with my mother. I told Brian I would just sneak on the bus with him, and he agreed. No one noticed as I slid in next to him on the bus. My mother must not have noticed either. I arrived with Brian and walked into his assigned classroom with him. The teacher asked us all to sit in a circle on the floor, and she began to call out names, asking us to raise our hands when we heard our name called. Obviously my name wasn't on the list, and when she was done, the teacher looked at me with a furrowed brow. After looking from me to my brother and comparing the freckles splashed on my cheeks and nose to the identical ones on my brother's face, it took her all of a minute to realize that I was Brian's sister. She asked me my name and how old I was. When I told her, she gasped and said, "Oh my, does your mother know where you are?" The look on my face was a dead giveaway. She let me sit down at a small, wooden table and gave me milk and graham crackers and told me that my mother was on her way to get me.

An hour or so later, my mother came rushing into the class, all melodramatic, and grabbed me, panting that she didn't know whether to hit me or hug me. She chose the hug option. I wasn't grounded or anything, and it ended up being a funny little story she would tell to everyone. I was just a fearless girl wanting to go to school.

Here I was, years later, about to embark upon a whole new schooling experience, and I was ecstatic, but this time full of fear—fear of failure, of not fitting in, of being stupid. I tried to push the fears out of the way and just focus on one task at a time. That made it much more bearable, because when I thought of it as a whole—like a whole class or a whole semester—I would get all in my head and scared again. I started slow, one step at a time. I was getting oriented to the campus and how to register for classes. I had to figure out a way to pay for it all, and I ended up filling out a million applications for every grant and loan I could find. I didn't want to have to work while in college because I knew this was going to take every ounce of brain power I had in me.

My parents agreed to help me with rent and bills while I was in college. My father was a working-class success, and in many ways didn't see the point of college. After all, he made an incredible living as a salesman for years without any additional schooling after high school, and he was damn proud of that. But my stepmother had gone to college and she fully understood the value of a college education. They both decided to support me in any way they could. I briefly looked into college dorms, and there was a "sober" dormitory, but I just didn't think it would be a good environment for me to be right on campus all the time. I needed the quiet solace my apartment offered me in order to maintain my recovery, and my parents agreed. It would be safer for me.

I realized quickly that college wasn't going to be easy. I had a lot of preparation work to do before I could even schedule classes. Because my GPA was so poor and I hadn't taken my SATs, I had to have testing done to determine my math and English skill level. I had never taken algebra or anything beyond that, so when I sat for this test, I felt like a moron. I had no idea what x equaled or how to determine a and b. I was lost, and my self-confidence plummeted to the industrial carpet below my desk. "Maybe I can't do this," I thought in the most self-defeating manner I had encountered since before I got into recovery. Was I crazy to think college was a viable option? I quickly shook the self-doubt out of my head and gave it my best try. I filled in the bubbles on the test knowing that I was simply guessing at the answers. I had heard once that C was always the safest choice on any multiple-choice test—I have no idea where I got this bit of brilliance, but I decided I would just start darkening all the Cs and randomly intersperse an A or B or D answer to make it look good.

I left the room feeling uneasy, but knowing somehow that it would all be okay.

23

HIGHER POWER

THIS WAS A NEW AND AMAZING FEELING THAT HAD
begun to take over in my life—that somehow, some way, I would be
okay. Feet planted, I saw a new pattern developing in my life. At that
point, my world was surrounded and embedded in my twelve-step
fellowship. This is common in early recovery. Life moves slower as we
begin to feel our way through each and every day with the newness of
recovery. It's always best to take things slow and not rush into anything.
I had spent two years in therapy dealing with all the reasons I used to
drink and drug. I was beginning to understand my own triggers and
demons and how to manage them to avoid old negative behaviors, or
worse, a relapse. I no longer had a desire to use or drink; the obsession
was lifted from me when I woke up in the hospital alive after my
suicide attempt. Now, thanks to a twelve-step program and going to
therapy, I was learning to deal with life on life's terms without picking

up a drink or drug. Instead I learned to deal, to feel, and to heal. It was important for me to keep my feet firmly planted in recovery.

The new positive pattern challenged my spiritual view in a good way. Good things were happening to me; things in my life were just working out somehow. I know a lot of it was due to my hard work and simply doing the footwork to get myself to the next step in my life, but there was more to it. Not only was I doing the footwork, but I was then letting it go and simply believing and trusting in the process.

I had begun praying a lot, which was also pretty new for me. I had always said foxhole prayers when I was using, like "God, just get me through this night and I will never do x, y, z again," or "God, please make the room stop spinning and I will never drink again." Often I was clinging to a toilet bowl when I had these false connections to God. My prayers now were different. They were less selfish, less about a pathetic plea negotiation and more about a working relationship.

I wasn't sure what my higher power was; I believed in God, but had no idea what exactly God was. However, I was willing to begin to trust and believe in this higher power, and the results in my life were proof that I was on the right track. Things just worked out for me. If I didn't have enough money to pay a bill, somehow, in some way, the money to pay the bill would find its way to me. Whether it would be a card from my parents with a check in it or a refund check from my insurance company, somehow things always managed to arrive just when I needed them. The universe began to provide for me.

I was in awe of this process because it had never existed in my life before. I began to really understand that in recovery, if I kept doing the next right thing, I would always get what I needed. I might not get what I wanted, but somehow, I would always get what I needed on any given day. It built a faith in me that became strong and foundational in my life. I had always heard in the rooms that one of the few requirements was to believe in a higher power of some kind, and I was fully embracing this concept.

The program doesn't attempt to define what your higher power must be; it just suggests that it is really important to have one. It makes sense to me. As addicts, we tend to be very self-centered people; after all, we thought we were in control of everything for so long. Many addicts walk with a godlike complex. Recovery is about getting out of yourself, out of your head, and realizing you're not in control and that you must rely upon others to succeed. It is a hard concept for many, but one that, if you don't complicate it too much, actually makes a lot of sense.

I've met people whose higher power was the rooms of their twelve-step fellowship. Or, as one old-timer in the rooms would say, his higher power's name was Ernie, and that was all he referred to him as—Ernie. It is that simple; he just believed in something greater than himself and it worked for him. Many people come into recovery with old baggage of God and church, so the thought of any form of religiosity in a program of recovery is enough to scare them right out of the process altogether. In my opinion, this is where the program is quite brilliant. It allows you to develop that relationship on your own and in a gentle manner.

I had often heard in meetings that there would come a time when the only thing that stood between me and my disease would be my higher power, so I had better harness that relationship and nurture it so I would be ready. It was beginning to make total sense to me, and the relationship I was starting to form with my not-yet-defined higher power felt nice and safe for me. It became something I could rely upon. The act of relying on something, of having faith in something, was brand-new to me. It felt stable, and for someone who had been as unstable as you can get, it was a blissful feeling.

My strength in recovery was solid. I was ready to take on more challenges and to grow into myself. With my foundation in recovery strong and my belief in a higher power in place, I knew I could get through any situation as long as I continued to live my life along the spiritual lines of the twelve-step program. I still spoke to my sponsor every day. I still went to meetings. However, my life became more than just twelve-step recovery. Especially with my entrance into college, it was also time for me to begin exploring more. So my life began to evolve and develop. I realized I could tackle more and more. More things came into my life and I found myself busier and busier. My life began to blossom, fill in the edges that once were rough, and make me whole. I knew how to handle situations that in the past would have left me broken. The twelve-step program was a bridge to a new life for me, and I didn't waste time standing on that bridge; I ran across it and embraced the life that awaited me on the other side.

24

FEELING SMART

A COUPLE OF WEEKS AFTER I'D TAKEN THE MATH TEST,
I received a letter in the mail that said I had failed it and needed to take
remedial math prior to taking a college-level course. I didn't get upset,
because I knew I hadn't done well on the test, and seriously, I was just
excited to be taking any classes. I had a thirst for knowledge that was
insatiable. I just wanted to start learning. I had neglected my brain for
so many years; it hadn't been really turned on since the sixth grade.
I hadn't taken any education seriously since that time, so I was ready
and eager to absorb everything that was coming my way. I scheduled
four classes, including English, Adolescent Development, the Remedial
Math course, and Sociology, at night since I was enrolled as a returning
adult student, which meant my courses were geared towards older
students and catered to the adult learning theory. This was perfect for
me. I was in class with other people my own age, and it gave me all day
to study and go to meetings.

Going to the bookstore and picking out my books was the most
exciting venture I'd had in a long time. Just walking through the
bookstore made me feel smart immediately, as if each book I passed
and touched was imprinting its knowledge upon me. When I stepped
onto campus, I had a sense of belonging that was solid. I felt like I
was right where I was supposed to be, and that feeling helped me glide
around in a state of wonderment like a small child entering Disney
World for the first time. I had to go get student identification, and as
I left the photo area with my new still-warm plastic badge in hand, I
stared at it in awe and felt like I was someone. The ID not only made
me feel like I had arrived at a new identity, but it made me feel like I
was coming home in some way. That little girl I abandoned so long
ago, the straight A-, perfect attendance-achieving girl that I left behind
in sixth grade was remerging inside of me, and the smile on my face
was just as magnificent as the feeling it produced inside me.

I remember coming home with my books and wanting to get a
jump start on my homework before my first class. I figured I better get
a nice lead since it had been so long since I had been in any form of
school setting, so I began to prepare my surroundings. Everything had
to be perfect; I had to create an environment conducive to learning.
I put sufficient lighting on, turned on a CD of sounds of nature to
gently float in the room, but not so loud as to distract my thinking
process. I lit several candles to create warmth and relaxation. I even
lit some incense to add positive energy and aroma. I wasn't messing
around; this was serious business! I pulled out my shiny new book,
a legal pad, a calculator I had just purchased—some big fancy thing
that was listed as a requirement—and my newly-sharpened pencil.
I was ready to tackle my first homework assignment. I surveyed my
surroundings and determined that I had in fact created the perfect
learning environment, and I felt good about diving into what was sure
to be a huge challenge. I was ready for anything and as organized as
I could have been. I knew how hard the math test had been, so I had
predetermined in my mind that this was going to be a struggle for

me. But I was up for the challenge, so I opened the book with great anticipation, but after seeing the first page I just burst out laughing. It was literally 2 + 2 and 4 + 4 and 6 + 6 and so on. All my expectations were shattered, and I was laughing so hard that tears were streaming off my face onto my perfect legal pad. I immediately picked up the phone and called my father, laughing so hard I almost peed my pants as I explained to him what my college homework actually entailed. We both found the humor and joy in this situation. Just like with everything else I was learning in this new life, I had to start at the bottom and work my way back up. Relearning all that I thought I had already learned was a big part of this process. It was fun, and needless to say, I got an A in that class. In fact, I got almost all A's that semester.

I adjusted rather well to college. I began going to noon meetings in town, which allowed me to mingle and mix with a different set of people in recovery. This was a good break from the lesbian crew, since Lynn was still giving me the silent treatment. I would still go to my Saturday morning meeting, and she would sit there with her arms crossed staring straight ahead the whole time. It hurt me that she was so angry with me, but I also knew there was nothing I could do about it, so I let her be and went about my new life. I loved going to school. I felt a part of something so much larger than myself when I stepped onto campus each day with my backpack strapped on. I loved the feel of walking to class with the rush of hundreds of students scurrying across campus from one class to another. I was a part of this energy and it made me feel confident in a new way. I began making friends in my classes, and I soaked in the environment.

25

UNEXPECTED THEATRICS

AFTER SPRING SEMESTER ENDED, I DECIDED TO TAKE
summer classes since I really had nothing else to do. These classes were
held during the day, which was different for me because I was so used
to going to night classes with older students. I had heard summer
classes weren't as hard. They were usually condensed due to the time
constraints of summer, and the class sizes were much smaller, so it
seemed to be a good idea to take a class I thought was going to be really
hard. So I scheduled another math course, this one nonremedial.

I enjoyed being on campus during the day—it made me feel more
like a "real" student, as opposed to this person who just snuck onto
campus at night. I once again restructured my meetings around my
classes. There were so many meetings in town that this was easy to
do, and it also forced me to mix up my meetings, which is always a
good thing to do in recovery. Sometimes going to the same meetings

over and over again can become a bit boring as ultimately you end up
hearing from the same people often. I made sure I was still making
at least four to five meetings a week. I knew that just because I was
starting to have this great new life, it was because of recovery that I
had it, and if I wanted to keep this new life, I needed to maintain my
attendance in meetings. It was hard balancing my schedule, my new
friends, and meetings, but I did it.

By that time I had decided to major in rehabilitation education,
because it seemed practical to become a drug and alcohol counselor
and try to help others. At that point in my recovery I hadn't quite come
into my own, and I was still very much in the mind-set that I had to
listen to others because my thinking wasn't always the best way to go. I
was trying to make the right decisions, the practical ones, and the ones
that made sense to the majority of those around me, as this was still a
part of my recovery process.

Originally I had wanted to major in communications and minor in
theater. Acting had always been something I wanted to pursue, and I
thought communications would be a great avenue for me. My parents
weren't too thrilled with my choices. My father didn't understand how
I could obtain a good job with those concentrations and worried that I
would struggle upon graduation. I took what he said into consideration,
even though my dreams were more in line with my first choice.

After meeting with my academic advisor, I knew I could complete
my degree in three and a half years as long as I didn't take any random
courses that didn't count. I knew I wanted to get my degree as quickly
as possible, so I was not going to take any courses that didn't fit into
my requirements for my major. In addition to the math class, I enrolled
in a theater class and was so excited to try out acting. I was only able
to take a certain number of electives and chose this class to be one of
them. I had always harbored a deep desire to be an actress; for whatever
reason, I just knew I would be a natural.

I had made a ritual out of watching award shows. I took them very seriously. I had rules: I had to be alone; a bowl of popcorn was my chosen dinner always (can't be bloated for the Oscars); and I had to have at least one bottle of wine, if not two, on standby. I would switch the program on in giddy anticipation. I loved watching the stars arriving in their glamorous outfits and walking the red carpet with such grace and style, all while waving like princesses at the adoring fans. I would practice my wave, my walk, and how I would stand and pose for pictures while saying, "Oh yes, isn't it lovely? It's Armani." I would guess the winner of each award and shout it out in eager delight as the presenter usually confirmed my assertion. Then I would stand, usually half in the bag at this point, holding my empty wine bottle as a microphone and droning my acceptance speech into my empty living room. It was all glam and drama, and I was drawn to that like butter to popcorn.

Just as I had suspected, even without the wine bottle mike, I was a natural in the class and fell in love with acting in a way I knew I would.

As summer gave way to fall, I started to see State College as my home. In Pennsylvania, fall is a breathtaking sight to see. Rolling hills quickly turn from bright, green patches of broccoli-like form to a virtual harvest of yellows, oranges, and reds. Leaves fell all around and swished and crunched under my feet as I zigzagged through campus from class to class. The brisk air felt incredible on my skin. It was my favorite type of weather, when jeans and a sweatshirt are the only reasonable choice and provide such incredible warmth that any thoughts of the summer sun on your skin are left far behind.

I felt I could stand tall and walk proud. I adjusted well to the day classes and decided to continue scheduling my classes that way. I wanted to fully embrace what being a student felt like. The energy on campus in the beginning of fall was amazing, all hustle and bustle, and I truly felt like a part of the college scene when I sat down in my first 200-person lecture. I made sure I sat up front at every class to ensure I paid attention. I knew I needed to in order to do well. The classes I took were fun and made me use parts of my brain that I hadn't accessed in years. I was getting good grades and enjoying the challenges.

One day I was sitting in biology class, listening attentively, when all of a sudden the walls around me began to close in and my breath got shallow. I didn't know what was happening to me, but my senses grew very sharp and my chest tightened. It reminded me of the night I took the ginkgo biloba. I quickly realized I was in the throes of a panic attack. I had to get out of the room. I somehow managed to get out of my seat, got down the hall, and slumped into a bathroom stall. I sat on the toilet with my mind spinning, trying to even my breathing and calm myself down. It was overwhelming. I was sweating. It hit me like a freight train, and intuitively I began to pray. I prayed the Serenity Prayer over and over again, asking for God's help. As I did, my pulse slowed, my breath returned to normal, and my shoulders lowered from my ears where they had taken up residence. I sat there for a couple of minutes, gathering myself. I felt exhausted.

I hated the panic attacks. I knew they were common for many in recovery, but I had only had that one the time I took the gingko biloba. It made me feel like I did when I used, which then left me feeling oddly remorseful, as though I *had* used—which I knew was crazy because I hadn't. It was my disease messing with me.

After I shared it with my sponsor and in a meeting that night, I was reassured that once again, it was just a normal part of recovery. Sometimes our disease pops up in random ways and takes over. It was one of those moments when it was just me and my higher power, and thankfully I had enough of a connection to calm myself down and get through the moment.

26

Flashback: Trauma and Blackout

I WAS BEGINNING TO HAVE PAIN IN MY BACK AND stomach. It would come on gradually and leave me feeling bloated. The pain was dull and constant. It felt like I couldn't have stretched my back enough to release the pain. I went to the health clinic on campus located in Ritenour Building, which was dubbed the "wait-an-hour" for its constant long line of ailing students with no health insurance waiting to be seen. After I waited more than an hour to be seen, the staff told me it was probably gas or indigestion and it would pass. Several more visits, X–rays, and an external ultrasound showed nothing.

As the first snow hit the ground, the pain persisted and got worse. I felt bloated all the time—like I had the worst case of PMS you could imagine. Several times it became so uncomfortable that I went to the emergency room in the local hospital. Each time I went, the doctors would push on my belly and tell me I had gas. This was beginning to annoy the shit out of me because I knew it wasn't gas. Gas doesn't last months. Every time, they attempted to give me a prescription for Vicodin to help ease the pain, and every time, I would politely remind the doctor that I was in recovery. By the third and fourth times, this was annoying me because I knew it was written down in my chart—I had insisted it be written down the second time they attempted to hand me a script. After the fourth time, I walked out of the ER. I was frustrated and confused and started to feel helpless. Every doctor I went to seemed like a past dealer trying to ignore the evidence that something was seriously wrong with me by simply medicating it. I tried to ignore it and cope with the pain, but it was so bad at times.

One night at a restaurant with some of my college friends, I doubled over in pain. They immediately rushed me to the hospital. When I was finally admitted, the doctors were once again baffled. One friend who was with me knew how frustrated I had been because of no one seriously helping me. So she became my medical advocate, demanding that I be seen and examined thoroughly while reminding them that I was in recovery and couldn't be given any narcotics. She was my guardian angel that day, the protector of my recovery. I was sore, tired, and traumatized.

The doctors once again wanted to send me home with a pain prescription and a diagnosis of gas. After my friend and I pleaded with them, insisting that I had more than gas, the doctors finally decided to perform an internal ultrasound on me.

The internal ultrasound was horrible. It was like being raped by Darth Vader. They take a large wand and put a huge condom over it, squish out some lube onto the tip, and insert the wand into your vagina. They then begin to thrust it around in there while pushing down on your stomach. It is horrifically humiliating and painful, and also retraumatizing for anyone who has ever been sexually violated. They should really attempt to get some form of sexual history from women before they do this procedure, because it could send the most rational of people into a pitfall of posttraumatic stress reactions. I focused on the popcorn ceiling and prayed quietly in my head, and after what seemed like hours of probing, the technician spotted some fluid on the screen and made the quick assessment that my appendix had burst and I needed immediate surgery to remove it.

I was rushed into a surgical room where people began swirling around me, taking blood, poking and prodding me in preparation for surgery. I was freaked out! I was pretty certain my appendix hadn't burst, even though I had no past experience to back up this hunch. I knew my problem was deeper; it was more chronic. But I was also relieved that a sense of urgency was finally surrounding me, because I had felt certain that something major was happening with me.

As they were rushing to get me into surgery, an aide was attempting to put an IV into my arm. I informed her that I had freakishly small veins and was historically a hard stick. She blew me off by saying that she was a professional. She was rude. I was pissed. She pricked me once, no go, and then twice, still nothing, then she wiggled the needle around in my arm until I screamed in pain. She was flustered. After the sixth plunge into my flesh, I'd had it. I screamed at the top of my lungs, "Get out!" as I pulled my sore, throbbing arm away from her grip. Her eyes widened and she rushed out of the room.

I knew I was out of hand, but I just couldn't stand one more needle stick into my bruised skin. All of this was too overwhelming. Everyone in the room came to an abrupt halt. I was shunned by the rest of the medical staff, and at that point I didn't care. Instead of all these strangers in white coats scurrying about, I just wanted my parents. I wanted someone who felt remotely loving around me, reassuring me that I was going to be okay.

A few minutes later my friend was at my side holding my hand and laughing quietly to herself. "You sure told that bitch," she said. I laughed as some of my tension eased.

Quickly another aide was brought in, and I could tell by her no-nonsense facial expression that she was here on business. She asked my friend to step aside and introduced herself and said she was there to try to get my IV in. I breathed in a huge, deep breath and looked away while she expertly slid in the IV. "See, that was no big deal, was it?" she asked. A tear ran down my cheek as I thanked her. I was exhausted by emotions. I asked to phone my parents, and when my dad picked up I began to sob. I told them I was being rushed into emergency surgery for what they thought was my appendix bursting. My parents were worried and asked me to call as soon as I could. My father had a big meeting scheduled the next day and wasn't able to come up right away. He assured me it was a very routine surgery that doctors do all the time and that I would be fine. I hung up feeling a little better.

My friend was told she had to leave the room while they prepped me for surgery. They mentioned the word *catheter,* and I freaked. I had never had one of those, but I'd heard they were really painful. They made me drink a huge bottle of a liquid that tasted like total crap to prepare me for the surgery, and I would need the catheter because I would apparently be eliminating this fluid while in surgery. I had already been violated by the ultrasound, and now they wanted to shove a tube up my urethra. I was traumatized, and it hurt like hell. They pushed a needle into my IV and said it would help calm me down. Within a couple of minutes, I felt my body loosen and felt a nice wave of calm come over me. The bright lights fuzzed a bit above me, and I watched all the nurses and aides swirl around me as they prepared me for surgery. Next thing I knew, I was being pushed out of the room and down a hall toward the surgical suite. The lights were brighter there, and it was colder. They told me they had to move me onto the long metal table in the middle of the room for the surgery. As they lifted me, I felt a tugging between my legs and an intense pain as they moved me, but not my catheter bag, off the table. I screamed out in pain, and the next thing I knew someone was holding the bag and another doctor was plunging another needle into my IV. Seconds later, blackness.

27

FLASHBACK: DRUGS AND THE C WORD

AFTER MY SURGERY, I HAD TO SPEND SEVEN DAYS IN
the hospital. I had more tubes coming out of my body than I had ever
seen—an IV, a catheter, and a tube that went up my nose, down my
throat, and into my stomach. The tube would pump excess junk from
my stomach out into a large machine next to my bed. My throat was
so sore. Everything hurt. Still not having any diagnosis only made
matters worse.

The doctor had come in the day after my surgery and told me they
had removed my appendix, and when they did, they found a large
abscess on my colon the size of a softball. They had to cut it out and
ended up removing a good portion of my colon as a result. He had no
idea what it was, but was thinking it might be some form of cancer.
I gasped. Just the word *cancer* sent me into flashbacks of holding my
mother as she lay lifeless after her own struggle from cancer. Cancer.

I rolled the word over in my brain in disbelief. Cancer at twenty-four. I began to freak out inside, thinking of how cancer had ravaged my mother's body and killed her. I started to cry hysterically. The doctor was cold. He knew nothing of me, nothing of my story, and he didn't understand. I felt so alone, and in that moment I wished my mother was there to comfort me. Instead I had a cold medical staff tending to me, and it only grew colder after the doctor left me with the word *cancer* hanging in the air like a death sentence. Just then, a stabbing pain hit my stomach. I hit the morphine button and everything went black.

I was abruptly awakened by a nurse who was checking my vitals. I was totally out of it, having been sleeping and filled with morphine. I opened my eyes and she said, in an extremely rude voice, "You really should try and get up. The longer you wait, the harder it will be." I was shocked. I had come out of surgery only hours ago and this nurse thought I should jump out of bed and walk around. My frustration fired up. I'd had enough of this staff; they were horrible. Forgetting the tube in my mouth, I barked back at her, but could barely talk and it just hurt more. I started crying so hard that my stomach ached from the contractions of my sobs. I was a mess. A throbbing was coming from between my legs, and my throat was killing me. I felt hopeless and defeated. For the second time in twenty-four hours, I screamed at someone and kicked her out of my room. I wasn't usually such a bitch, but these people had zero sympathy at a time when I needed buckets of it.

I was also very much under the influence of the morphine that kept sinking into my veins, which made everything around me fuzzy. I reached for the phone, barely noticing that it was 2:00 a.m., and I dialed my parents' phone. By the time I heard my father's sleepy voice pick up, I was nearly hysterical, so I just softly babbled and begged for them to please come and get me and take me home. I could barely talk, but I managed to say that the staff was horrible, and my nurse was like Nurse Ratched from the movie *One Flew Over the Cuckoo's Nest.* That made my father laugh. The sound of his laughter put me at ease a bit as he tried to reassure me once again that I would be fine and I should just try and get some sleep. They would be coming in a day or two. I hung up realizing I hadn't told him about the cancer. I pushed the button on the morphine again and went back to sleep.

I woke up the next day with a very dry and horrible taste in my mouth. The tube hurt so badly that I cried almost every hour. I could only have ice chips, and those were few and far between, so that my stomach would heal. Seconds after I would suck on an ice cube, I would see black fluid fly up the tube from my stomach, through my nose, and into the machine. It was both horrifying and amusing. It became a little trick I would do for everyone who came to visit me.

I was also still hooked up to a morphine drip, which freaked me out. The first day or two, I hit that button like the good addict I was. I was in pain. My abdomen had just been torn open. I needed it. But by day three, as I started to become more aware and mobile, I started to feel weird about it. My recovery instincts kicked in, and I asked for its removal. I explained to the doctor that I was in recovery and felt it was no longer needed. He eyed me skeptically, but respected my decision and ensured me that if I was in pain, I could immediately call the nurse and get some Vicodin. I told him that would not be necessary. I was never a pill popper in my addiction history, but I was smart enough to know that a drug is a drug and that I have an addiction. I didn't want anything to jeopardize my recovery.

The thought of losing the time I had built up in recovery crushed my chest inward in a way that was more painful than the staples in my stomach. I couldn't imagine myself having to walk back into the rooms of recovery and get a twenty-four-hour chip again, or looking my new friends in the eye and knowing I had let them down. The thought of my parents' disappointment was too much for me to bear. And lastly, the idea of letting my new higher power down in that way was intense for me. I was still in the process of figuring out what my higher power was, but on a daily basis I was praying to my God. I could not handle the idea of turning my back on God again as I had done so often in my addiction. My mind had been too informed at this point in recovery to throw it all away. I had a new definition of pride and ego in recovery, and they were strong protectors of my new way of life.

Even though my parents weren't there yet, I certainly wasn't lonely; my new family showed up in droves. Many of my friends in recovery poured into my hospital room over the next seven days, and I was amazed by the unconditional love and support I received from those in the program. Lynn didn't come to see me; she was still too pissed off at me for breaking her heart. I secretly wished she had come.

I had only been in State College for a little over a year, but I had more flowers in my room than a new mother living in the community her whole life. The nicer nurses kept making comments about the overflow of cards and flowers and the constant stream of people in and out of my room. I had never had so many people truly and genuinely care about me in this way. I kept being amazed at the depth of love and support that existed in the rooms of recovery. I could count on so many people to be there when I needed them. In my using life, I was lucky if I could count on a handful of people, and usually only if there was something in it for the other person would a hand be extended. This was free and unconditional support, and it made me glow like a toddler at a birthday party in awe of all the presents.

The expressions of concern and support I received were overwhelming and literally gave me the high I needed to dull the pain. I felt more love in those days and more of a sense of family and home than I had ever felt my whole life. It reaffirmed for me that I was indeed in the exact place I was supposed to be in my life. State College was home in every sense of the word.

28

RELEASE, FINALLY

MY PARENTS CAME AND WERE A HUGE HELP FOR ME IN getting me back into my apartment and settled. They were amazing. They hung out with me in the hospital much of the time. When they weren't visiting with me, my stepmother was scrubbing my apartment clean and caring for my cat. She is hands-down the most organized person I know. We used to joke at home that if you were cooking in the kitchen and turned your back on a pot, she would have it cleaned and in the dishwasher before you turned back around. She taught me how to organize myself and my life, how to keep a clean house, and how to take care of my things. She taught me how to be a productive and high-functioning woman in so many ways. As she began to comment on my new actions in recovery, it was an honor for me to be able to show her the life lessons she had instilled in me.

I told them what the doctor had said about not knowing what it was they had removed from me, and about the possibility of cancer. The doctor hadn't been back since, so I was left each night to sit and ponder what this all meant for me. I knew in my heart that if I truly did have cancer, I would fight it like hell. I wouldn't just succumb to it the way I felt that my mother had. I would suit up for battle and it would be on. I was just starting to live my life, and there was no way I was going to let something come in and kill me now, not after I had fought so hard this year for this new life.

Finally, on the fourth day, my feeding tube and catheter were removed. A new nurse gently tugged the tube out of my scratchy, sore throat and liberated me, which felt like heaven. I could breathe again without pain, and better yet, I could have a real drink of water. After the way the catheter had almost been ripped out of me on the way to the surgery table, this time I braced for sheer hell. My parents left the room. As the nurse pulled the catheter out, it stung a bit, but once it was out I was so happy I peed a little on the sheets. Now not only was I liberated from the tubes, but this meant I could attempt to get out of bed. In fact, I was being forced to stand up because the nurse had to change my sheets. I felt extremely wobbly and clung to the wall while she quickly remade my bed, and then I gladly slid back under the sheets.

Later that day, after much probing and persistence from my father, the doctor reemerged with great news. He told me I did not have cancer. A rush of relief flooded over me and tears began to roll down my checks. I saw my parents' eyes fill up a bit too. The relief in the room was palpable. He went on to say I had a condition called diverticulitis. He explained that diverticulitis is a condition in which little pockets that form in the colon suddenly rupture. The rupture results in infection in the tissues that surround the colon. He explained that my rupture led to infection, which often clears up after a few days of treatment with antibiotics, but since I was never properly diagnosed, the infection worsened and the softball-sized abscess formed in the wall of the colon and began leaking toxic waste into my body. He said I would have most likely died had I not come into the emergency room when I did.

Those words really hit me hard as my eyes widened. I almost died—again, within a little over a year. Except this time it was not by my own hands. I was dumbfounded, and incredibly grateful for my friend who insisted to the medical staff that I be checked out thoroughly. Had it been up to the ER staff, I would have been discharged with a diagnosis of gas and a prescription for Vicodin.

The doctor said it was odd that I had this condition, because it is mostly found in people much older than I was. I sat quietly, wondering if all the laxatives I ate like candy in high school to keep my weight down had anything to do with my current condition. I was afraid to ask, having never really spoken in front of my parents about my eating disorder in the past. I was pretty sure they knew about it since every time I ate with them, I was in the bathroom moments later. I took a deep breath and just asked. The doctor absorbed the information for a minute, and I watched my parents sit still as boards, doing the same. He said it could have been, but there was no real medical way to determine if that was the cause. It was enough for me, however, to vow to never, ever take a laxative again. After rehab, I took my recovery seriously enough to realize that bingeing and purging were not part of a healthy lifestyle.

The doctor said I would have to seriously watch my diet—to not eat things with seeds and try to take in more fiber—which I knew was going to be a little hard living on a college student budget and having fast food all around me. I was to follow up with a doctor periodically for checkups. I did the follow-up appointments, and after that I had no problems again. I would often still eat cashews and popcorn, items traditionally on the do-not-eat list, but I didn't get sick again.

The air in the room lightened up after he left. We all just kind of looked at each other in relief after all the information that had been exchanged: cancer, nearly died, eating disorder. Before we had a chance to discuss any of it, Nurse Ratched came in. I signaled to my dad with my eyes that she was the one. He smiled. She was her usual cranky self as she checked my vitals.

She told me once again that I should try to move around and walk around, which felt like the last thing on earth I wanted to do. With an incision that was three and a half inches long, my every move hurt like hell. On the sixth day, I was informed that I would not be able to leave the hospital until I farted. Yes, until I passed some good old-fashioned gas. Apparently that would be the hospital's scientific guarantee that my system was functioning properly and that I was well enough to be shipped home. Never in my life did I want to rip one so badly. I began walking the halls of the hospital because I had been instructed that movement helps with the passing of gas.

Finally, on the morning of day seven, it happened: I was sitting with my parents and we were joking about something, and in the middle of a good, hard, and painful belly laugh, a little toot slipped out from under my hospital gown. We all cheered like it was the fourth of July! I called the nurse as though I was calling in the winning numbers of the lottery. When Nurse Ratched walked in the room, I exclaimed, "I farted!" She wasn't very amused. She nodded, gave me a nice, fake smile, and said, "I'll inform the doctor and begin your discharge papers. You can go home today." She walked out and we all burst into laughter. I was so excited to go home, finally!

29

FLYING OUT OF THE CLOSET

I WALKED INTO MY HOME TO FIND MY CAT PURRING
and circling my ankles like crazy, obviously pleased to see me home
at last. My whole body was instantly warmed with the unconditional
love my cat spun around my ankles, and it rose to fill my heart. Home
never felt sweeter. My parents helped me get settled in and made sure
I had everything I needed for the weeks to follow. I was to rest and
heal for the next four weeks—no school or anything else but staying
home and recuperating. I was concerned about my classes and what
this would do to my grades, but I also knew that I had to take care of
myself first and the rest would fall into place.

My parents hung out with me for a little while and then went
on their way back home. They had a four-hour drive ahead of them.
I thanked them for everything as they left. It wasn't until later that I
would realize how much they did for me while I was in the hospital.

In the bathroom I found cleaning items, bags of kitty litter and food, and a ton of toilet paper. In the kitchen there were paper towels under the sink, and when I opened my cabinets, I found all the foods and snacks I loved so much—Doritos, cashews, and popcorn. As I moved on to the refrigerator, I found more of my favorites—Diet Pepsi, juice, cheese, ice cream. My heart swelled with gratitude as tears came to my eyes.

As I held a bottle of my favorite flavored creamer for my morning coffee, I felt like the luckiest girl alive. My parents loved me and provided for me in such an amazing way, and I knew it was because I was finally deserving of it all; I was finally showing up for life and living in a way that made them proud. Even though these waves of emotion were becoming familiar to me by now, on this particular day I found myself overwhelmed and exhausted with sentiment. I sobbed quietly, tears of joy and sadness flooding down my cheeks as I stood in front of the refrigerator. Maybe it was the combination of brushing with death and the parental nurturing that hit me in that moment. I was in awe of how different my life was, but then my stomach began to ache, so after pulling myself together I moved into my living room and cautiously set up camp. It hurt to bend and move too much, and I knew just going from the hospital to home had wiped me out both physically and, now, emotionally.

I carefully pulled my futon into its down position and placed my pillows and comforter from my bed. As I slid under the comforter, my cat curled up beside me. This would be my resting place for the next couple of weeks, and I was okay with the idea of just chilling for a while. I hadn't really sat still since I had moved into this apartment; I was running off to meetings, emotionally breaking down in therapy, entering into challenging, emotional, confusing relationships, and starting college all at once. It was nice to have an excuse to just stop. I drifted off to sleep, the warmth of my cat against my stitches somehow easing the pain.

I spent the next couple of days entertaining visits from my friends in recovery, playing games, and watching movies. While the visits were great for my spirits, I swore the laughter would kill me with stomach pain. But it was worth it. It offered a level of healing and pain relief that no pill could produce. I was not taking any of the pain medications they tried to give me when I left—I wasn't comfortable with the idea of taking narcotics at home. It was different while I was in the hospital after the first couple days of my recovery from surgery. The pain was there, but it wasn't as if I was going to die from it; that I knew. So I toughed it out the rest of the way and it really wasn't that bad. I had fifteen metal stitches going across the right side of my abdomen, and they were sore, but not unbearable. Actually they were kind of cool, and every time someone came over, I proudly lifted my shirt so show off my new metal. I already had my belly button and my tongue pierced, along with nine other holes in my ears left over from my teenage years, so this was just like an addition to my collection for me to flaunt.

My friend Brenda came by with a movie she had just rented and asked if I wanted to borrow it. It was an all-lesbian movie about a group of college friends who reunite years later after one couple has a baby—kind of like a lesbian *Big Chill*. I was intrigued. Brenda had watched me go through the whole saga of my latest relationship and my uncertainty about my sexuality. I eyed the movie cover suspiciously. I had never watched a lesbian movie before. The only lesbian scenes in movies I had ever seen were gratuitous shots of hot chicks making out briefly for the pleasure of a guy, like in *Cruel Intentions* or *Wild Things*.

After Brenda left, I popped some popcorn and settled in to watch the movie. As the characters came to life and the story arc built in the movie, I was entranced. I found myself nodding frantically in acknowledgment of what the characters were saying and laughing out loud at all the inside jokes like I somehow knew everyone, because somewhere deep down, I did. I got it. I knew it and I felt it. In the pit of my stomach, an understanding of and affiliation with these women awoke inside me. I loved every minute of their interactions and found myself feeling connected to them in such a comfortable and natural way. All at once, realization hit. I sat up and said aloud, "Oh my god, I'm gay!"

Just like that, I finally made the acknowledgment that had haunted me since kindergarten and stayed with me, buried deep down, throughout my entire life up until this point. I wasn't bisexual and I certainly wasn't straight. I was as gay as the day was long, and suddenly I just *knew* it and embraced it. All the past fears and denial that I allowed to crowd my head, heart, and soul just poured away from me as I sat in this profound awakening. I was finally fully and totally free. I was sort of in shock and immediately picked up the phone and dialed Brenda. I was so excited and elated that before she even said hello, I screamed out, "Brenda, I am gay!" I rambled on and on about how I couldn't believe it had taken me this long to finally acknowledge something that was so clear and present to me in this moment. She just softly chuckled and said, "So I take it you liked the movie." I just laughed so hard that I began to cry.

As the days went by and I was slowly becoming more and more comfortable walking around, I began to resume my daily life. I went back to meetings and planned my schedule for starting back to school. As I embarked on each step back into the real world, there was a new strength in my walk, a new certainty in my movement that felt so incredibly true. I felt like me in a way that I had never known. It was as though all the pieces that were scattered around in my soul came together all at once, and I knew without any doubt that this is exactly who I always was and was meant to be. I felt whole and real. I felt solid and completely grounded in myself for the first time in my life. This is who I am; I am a gay woman.

The acknowledgment of this kept growing inside me with every breath I took, and each breath of this truth filled me to perfection. I began telling everyone I knew in my meetings. "I am gay" came floating out of my mouth with such pride and ease to everyone I encountered over the next couple of days and weeks. Most of them were not surprised by this—it was pretty evident in my growth process that this was most likely the path I was heading down. But none of my recovery friends made assumptions or judgments upon me, they just simply let me be me and become me in a truly and wonderfully unconditional way. A couple of my male friends were a little taken aback; they had just assumed my pseudo-relationship was a phase. I knew this was no phase—it was just the opposite. It was the completion of something I had known forever.

I am. I finally knew who I was, and this declaration made me rise higher than I had ever gone with any drug or drink. It solidified the concrete foundation I was already crafting for myself in recovery. I am!

30

Buses and Butterflies

A NEW SEMESTER WAS RIGHT AROUND THE CORNER, and I was ready to head back to school after having the metal stitches removed from my abdomen. My car had broken down and finally died. I wasn't surprised—I had gotten more than my full share of usage out of the 1985 Toyota. However, it did mean that I was without transportation, which I wasn't too thrilled about. I didn't have money for another car and my parents were in no position to purchase one for me, so I was left with one humbling alternative: mass transit. I had never lived in a city, so I wasn't used to taking buses to my destinations. Since age seventeen, I had always had a car.

Fortunately for me, State College caters to students, so buses ran all over town every ten minutes. Conveniently, there was a bus stop at the top of the entrance to my apartment complex. I purchased my first bus pass and quickly learned how to navigate the bus system. It actually wasn't bad at all, except when I wanted to quickly run to the store and grab something. On the bright side, there were no more worries about parking tickets on campus or downtown fights for a parking place. I had racked up a couple of parking tickets in the past, and couldn't afford them on my limited budget anyway. It also added more structure to my life; I had to schedule my day a bit more, around the bus schedules and stops. I saved money on gas, but it meant my trips home to Allentown would now be limited to the bus system, which was okay because I was now finding myself going home only on semester breaks.

I was excited to get back into the swing of things on campus. I did some online research, trying to find some resources for my newfound gay identity. I knew I wanted to get involved and start meeting other gay women my own age. While I loved the group of women I hung out with in recovery, they were all much older than I was, and since I had already tapped into a little drama with my pseudo-relationship, I decided it was time to start finding people closer to my own age in college to relate to. The prospect of meeting other young, gay women excited me. I came upon a support group on campus for newly out or questioning females, and I figured that would be as good as any place to start. I e-mailed the person in charge to express my interest, and a day later I found an e-mail in my inbox from her telling me all about the group and when they met.

The premise of the group was to bring together women who were questioning their sexuality in a safe and emotionally healthy environment. With much anticipation, I walked up to the building where the group was to meet. I felt as though I were seeing campus in a whole new way as the new me, and it was thrilling. I was careful in picking out my outfit that night; after all, I had no idea what the new, gay me was going to look like. I had already begun vastly altering my appearance just based on my own growing sense of self, but now with this "gay" identifier, I didn't know what I was supposed to wear. My hair was still long to my shoulders and bleached blonde, hiding my natural, much darker, brown hair color peeking out from my roots.

My weight was down considerably thanks to my surgery, so all of my jeans were super-baggy. I had lost fifteen pounds! I wore a pair of jeans and a blue sweater that brought out the color of my eyes.

As I approached the building, I was nervous. I noticed a petite, bald girl with glasses wearing an oversized, red hooded sweatshirt and standing by the door, and I knew instantly that she was there for the group. Suddenly I felt vulnerable and scared as I stood in front of her. I managed to mutter out a few sentences, something like "Are you here for the ummm, you know, the ummm, group?" She smiled widely and said, "Yes. My name is Cassie and I come here often." I laughed as the tension fell into my socks. Her smile was so sweet and inviting that I immediately felt at ease. I introduced myself and told her this was my first time, which was about as obvious as the fact that we were standing there together. She guided me into the building and up a couple of flights of steps.

We were in the counseling building on campus because the group was led by a psychiatrist. The room was small, with two couches and some wooden therapy-style chairs in a circle. It felt comfortable because I had been spending most of my time in recovery rooms with a similar setup these days. There were already two other girls sitting there when we walked in, and Cassie gladly introduced me to both of them. Danielle and Mary were their names. They were both similar to me, and I was struck by how alike we seemed. They, too, had long, blonde hair and were on the "pretty girl" side, unlike my new friend Cassie with her shaved head and bulky sweatshirt. Cassie had that clear "I'm a dyke" persona, while the other two girls I wouldn't have picked out in a million years. I guess I had a real stereotypical image of what lesbians looked like, although that was now challenged every time I stared into a mirror. I was relieved to see that I wouldn't be the only "femme" girl in the group.

As we all made small talk, a couple of other women entered the room, and then the group leader and another woman came in, closed the door, and sat down. The psychiatrist was much older, so I identified her right away. She was a nice-looking butch woman, and my heart began to pound just a little louder inside my chest as she opened her mouth and began to introduce herself and everyone else. It was clear to me in that moment that I liked the more butch women. My pulse quickened just a little bit more around them.

Which is the total opposite of any woman I had been attracted to in my past encounters. When I was using, I was always experimental. Having known all my life that I had an attraction for women, it seemed to come out more when I was drinking. I always went toward feminine women, probably because that was all I had to choose from. I used to make out with my best friend all the time when we were loaded, and she is more feminine that I am. I had one lesbian sexual encounter in my addiction, but it came in the form of a threesome with a boyfriend on my twenty-second birthday. It was a blur because I was drunk as usual. All I really remember is being at the bar with my boyfriend, and when he asked me what I wanted for my birthday, I pointed at a hot blonde and said, "Her." It certainly wasn't a memorable evening. When it surfaced in my mind, I only felt shame and remorse. Like with other drunken sexual encounters I'd had in my addiction, I didn't like to think about it. They were just painful reminders of how low I had sunk.

Since I was taking my classes during the day now, I started spending more of my nights on campus instead of hanging out with my recovery friends. I was still going to meetings, but I was trading my late nights at Denny's for all things gay on campus. I got some flak from my younger twelve-step crew, but I was evolving a different way, and with Lynn still being so weird with me, it was a nice break from my older lesbian crew. So I began hanging out with my new lesbian friends from the campus support group, and they introduced me to the gay world on campus. I couldn't believe there were so many groups and activities to get involved in. Pride Week, an annual week of celebration of all things queer, was coming up and there was a slew of events on campus to attend. The prospect of going and mingling with a bunch of other gay people was so exciting to me because I knew I was ready to really try out my new identity. I was ready to have a gay experience without alcohol or drugs.

31

PROUD AND IN LOVE

THE SAME WEEK I ATTENDED THE LESBIAN SUPPORT group, I went to my first gay pride rally. It was empowering and exhilarating to be around so many out and proud young gay people. Most of the students looked rather stereotypically gay. The women all had short hair and adorned their backpacks with rainbows and buttons with empowering and funny slogans like "I'm not a lesbian but my girlfriend is." I felt slightly awkward because I still didn't know what my gay identity looked like on the outside. The one thing I did know was that the minute I was around these gay women, I felt like I belonged, and that this group of people whom I could identify with so naturally and easily had just been waiting for me to arrive. It's the same way I always felt when I walked into a recovery meeting, as if I was home and it was just—right.

As I walked up to the information table to check out the various on-campus resources, I was brought to a halt by a smile so captivating that my whole body just froze. As I soaked in the image, the most beautiful face I had ever seen came into focus. Her full lips formed a smile that extended across her face like a burst of sunshine. It was almost too hard to look at, but I found my eyes glued to her face. She had super-short, shiny black, spiky hair, and while her look screamed "dyke," she was soft around the edges. She had femininity within her masculine appearance and that immediately intrigued me. Before I realized it, she had shifted her gaze in my direction and sent a ray of sunshine out of her mouth in the form of a hello, and instead of responding in kind, I just stared blankly at her with what had to have been the dumbest look on my face. Quickly my friend Cassie interjected an introduction. "Jennifer, this is Raye. Raye, this is Jennifer." My mouth still had no ability to form any type of sentence, and I said nothing as a blush formed on her cheeks. I felt even more stupid about my lack of action until her smile grew even wider. At that point I was certain I blushed harder than I ever had in my life, and finally I managed a hello. Before I realized it, Cassie pulled me away while someone else grabbed Raye's attention. Cassie was laughing hard as I let out a huge breath of air, and it wasn't until then that I realized I had been holding my breath. This outburst just made Cassie laugh even harder as she said, "Raye tends to have that effect on some girls." I felt warm the rest of the day as I kept her smile in the forefront of my mind.

After that, I went to a meeting and shared about my experiences that day. I had always been brutally honest when sharing in meetings. I knew that was a cornerstone of my staying clean and sober, and I wasn't about to change that now. I had begun speaking freely in my meetings about my new identity, and while at first I was nervous and not sure how some people would respond, I knew I was in a safe place and that I had to express myself. There were no secrets anymore in my recovery, ever! Most people just got a kick out of me, the newcomer who was just discovering herself. I would elicit lots of laughter, and I didn't know if they were laughing with me or at me, but I didn't care because I was full of joy. I look at those same newcomers who come into meetings today and just chuckle, because I so understand the level of excitement they are experiencing. Early recovery is such a exploration; at times it can be painful when you are working your program properly, but then there are the times when you are so fiercely alive in your own skin that you cannot contain yourself. This is how I felt that day, and in the meeting as I shared, I knew I was practically exploding with anticipation and excitement and everything I was feeling inside.

Later that night, I walked into the dark room and felt an odd familiarity. Strobe lights glistened from the ceiling, casting shards of speckled light across the floor and splashing the bodies dancing to house music that was thumping from the DJ booth in the corner of the room. A tinge of panic rose in my stomach as memories surfaced of the old days of walking into club after club. It was still hard for me at times to be in environments that could serve as a trigger for me. Old memories would surface, and they challenged my foundation and strength in early recovery. I would have to talk myself down in my mind, telling myself that I was safe and it was okay because that wasn't my life anymore. These were always the times when I found the Serenity Prayer to be incredibly useful. Just repeating it over and over in my mind, while taking deep cleansing breaths, would remove the anxiety from me. I did this in my head as I walked into the room.

Cassie was all smiles as she waved me into the room. I reminded myself that this was not a bar or nightclub, but a college dance. I shook off the panic and followed her enthusiastic lead. All around me were small groups of students gathered together, people watching or paired off dancing. There were bright, rainbow-colored balloons clustered and scattered throughout the room and several round tables with chairs off to the side. The room reminded me of the high school dances I used to attend, and in a way I felt just as I had back then—all nerves and hormones raging in anticipation of what the night would bring. Of course, back then I would have been half-loaded, as I was sure many of these folks were, but if they were it wasn't obvious.

Out of the corner of my eye, I caught a glimpse of a girl with her arms tangled up in another girl, and I stopped dead in my tracks. It was her—Raye—and when she saw me, a smile broke across her face once again. She waved, and I waved back as the girl she was holding just looked from my face to hers with a question clearly on the tip of her tongue.

I pulled away my gaze and rushed up to Cassie, bursting with a million questions. Cassie filled me in that Raye had a girlfriend. I stole another glance in Raye's direction and said, "I am going to marry that girl." Cassie just laughed and said, "Get in line, honey."

32

FIREWORKS

AFTER THAT NIGHT I FELT ELECTRIC, LIKE I HAD A NEW window into my future, and it gave me such a jolt that I almost didn't need a cup of coffee to get up in the morning. Everywhere I went on campus, I looked for her, hoping for a glimpse of that amazing smile. I started going to as many gay-related meetings on campus as I could.

I joined the Lambda Student Alliance, a group for queer students that focused on education, awareness, and political events on campus. It was there at my first meeting that I would meet people who would shape my life for the coming years, including one who became my steadfast mentor, the group's advisor, Dr. Sue Rankin. She was an older butch lesbian with whom I immediately found solace, friendship, and guidance. She and I had a wonderful connection. She saw me as a young and energetic lesbian, new to the gay world, and she made it her job to gracefully walk me through all the changes that I would go through over my years at college.

Cassie had also told me about a lesbian sorority on campus and that immediately intrigued me, especially after she told me that Raye was a sister. I wanted in!

I had a lot of preconceived notions about sororities and what they stood for, and every single one I had was about to be challenged significantly as I readied myself to attend my first Lambda Delta Lambda (LDL) party.

The sorority consisted of about forty women, and at that time about five of them shared a house downtown at 507 Atherton Street, but everyone just called the joint "507." They certainly were not the über-feminine type of sorority sisters one would think of with long, cascading blonde hair. They were all thicker than your average stick-skinny sorority sister stereotype, and most of them had super-short, spiky hair. They wore baggy clothes and had that "just got out of bed" look perfected. They had style that seemed effortless but that you knew took them time in front of the mirror. I felt comfortable with them as soon as I walked in.

On my way to the sorority party, I made sure I stopped at the gas station on the corner and purchased some green tea to take with me. I had learned from my past experiences to have my own drink in hand at all times in situations where alcohol was present to avoid the "Can I get you a drink?" or "Why don't you have a drink?" questions that would be sure to come. The sisters were great about my decision not to drink; they were proud of the way I had changed my life. Never did any of them make me feel bad about not drinking, which was a welcome feeling.

During the party, I saw Raye in the corner of the room and our eyes met. She excused herself from the conversation she was carrying on and confidently walked toward me and said hello. I was so nervous to speak to her. I didn't know what I would say, but even as the panic rose in my throat, words came out of my mouth with a casual ease that took me off guard. We began the usual get-to-know-you kind of talk, and before I knew it hours had passed and Raye and I had held court in the corner of the room, talking nonstop. I couldn't believe how easy it was to talk with her and how comfortable I felt in her presence, even though when our eyes met the electricity was so intense that I had to look elsewhere. I had never felt such exhilaration when looking into another's eyes before, and it both energized me and scared the shit out of me.

It was getting late, and I knew I had to catch the bus to get home. Raye didn't have a car either, but said she would walk me to the bus stop and wait with me. I thought this was incredibly chivalrous. We made small talk as we made our way through campus in the dark to the bus stop in front of the student union building. I had successfully managed to avoid my past during our talks at the party. It wasn't hard, because we mainly focused on the present, what courses we were each taking, what the sorority was like, who was sleeping with whom. She had filled me in on all the up-to-date information on each sister and familiarized me with all of them.

But as we sat alone, with no distractions around us, the conversation took an inevitable turn toward me. She began asking more pointed questions, and before I knew it, I was spilling my guts to her. It was like water flowing out of my mouth; my deepest, darkest secrets spilled out with ease. I felt so incredibly comfortable with this woman that nothing I said held its usual hesitance or hidden fears. I trusted her implicitly, and more importantly, I trusted myself enough to know that this was my life and it was okay to lay it bare to whomever would be entering my life, whether it be as a friend or more than a friend. I was used to telling my story to those in recovery. It was kind of exciting to be speaking to someone who really had no understanding of recovery. She just sat there, holding intently to the words coming out of my mouth. I could see the intrigue and, at times, disbelief in her eyes when I got to the hard parts—the suicide attempt, the death of my mother, rehab. She never wavered, though; there was no disgust or judgment in her voice when she asked more questions or when she would just nod with incredible sympathy.

As I spoke, bus after bus came and went, and neither of us broke from the conversation. She could have had an easy out if she had been concerned about what I was telling her by just saying, "Hey, isn't that your bus?" But she didn't. Eventually, I glanced at my watch and realized there would only be one more bus coming to that stop for the night. I gushed about how I couldn't believe I had rambled on for so long and thanked her profusely for listening to me. She just smiled her amazing smile at me and said it was her pleasure. She thanked me for sharing with her. As my bus pulled up, I didn't want to get on. I didn't want the night to end. We just looked at each other, and I handed her my e-mail address and phone number. She said she'd call, and as I sank into my seat on the bus, I knew she would. I watched her smiling face grow smaller and smaller as the bus drove away, and I felt like I was floating above the bus with glee. I was in love and I knew it. I barely knew this person, but I loved her and I felt it in every fiber of my being, from the tingle in my toes to the warmth around my heart. I laid my head down that night and dreamt of her. She called the next day, and we made plans to go on a date. A date! With a girl. But not just any girl. With Raye! I was beside myself.

This was huge to me. I had just found a new group of friends that I knew I would cherish. I decided to pledge the sorority. And I had met and fallen in love with Raye. I had anxiety and butterflies lingering in my stomach, so I called my sponsor Rose for guidance.

Rose wasn't as thrilled for me.

As I had begun to grow in my recovery and take on college, she and I had begun to pull apart a bit. It wasn't that she wasn't a great sponsor; it just seemed like our lives were going in such different directions that there was a tension between us now. She had been such a strong support person for me whom I spoke to daily and told everything to; but this started to feel odd, and I began to feel uncomfortable speaking about my sexuality with her, because she wasn't really out of the closet. Even though we all knew she was gay, she had never had an actual experience with another woman and therefore never confirmed or denied her feelings. After I made my announcement and confirmation that I was gay, that was when the tension in our conversations and relationship began. I can only surmise that she had a discomfort with my newfound gay identity that I wore so freely, while hers was still tucked away, semi-hidden. She was cold when I talked about Raye, and my excitement was met with concern on her part that I was rushing into something and that I needed to focus on recovery. The unconditional support that I had come to rely upon was replaced with consternation and a bit of resentment.

As I hung up the phone, I realized that it might have been time to find a new sponsor. I was upset because I didn't like confrontation at all, and the last thing in the world I wanted to do was to disappoint or hurt her. It isn't uncommon in recovery to have a series of sponsors throughout your time. Rose was wonderful and really gave me what I needed in the beginning of my recovery, but as I began to grow spiritually and educationally, she didn't seem to fit my life anymore. I think I simply outgrew her. This happens in recovery. People can surpass others in terms of growth. It doesn't mean I was better at recovery than her or that I was in some way more evolved; it was just that I was moving in a different direction than her in my recovery and she was no longer the right guide for me through my journey.

I knew I would have to start seeking out a new sponsor, and I made a mental note of it as I readied myself for my date with Raye. She was taking me to the Grange Fair, an annual event on the outskirts of State College. Raye grew up in State College and was an agriculture major. While Pennsylvania State University was a rather progressive institution, it was embedded in a vast rural area of central Pennsylvania. The Grange Fair consisted of entertainment, agricultural competitions, attractions, truck and tractor pulls, crafts, rides, a circus, music, food, and more. It was historically and culturally important to the community and attracted thousands of people every year who camped in tents and recreational vehicles during the week-long event for which the school year was delayed so families could attend.

Raye's cousin had an RV and camped there every year with her family. Raye had borrowed her father's car and picked me up and told me all about the fair as we drove. We had a blast at the fair; we played games and laughed as every one of my white, plastic balls bounced off the rims of the glass bowls containing fish, while hers splashed directly into the water. We shared a huge funnel cake with cherry topping and whipped cream—it was about a thousand calories, and we devoured it together. I didn't even like cherry sauce, but I couldn't remember anything tasting as sweet.

It was the perfect date, only made better on the drive home when she pulled off the long, windy dirt road up to a large lake surrounded by trees in full fall foliage. We got out of the car as the sun was setting, and it was a breathtaking sight. I took it all in as the fall air was turning from day to night and the sky was growing dark. A shiver ran down my body as Raye reached for my waist and pulled me toward her. She was leaning up against the car, and as my body caved into hers and our lips met, my whole body lit up like a firefly in the night. As we parted lips, she looked up to the sky; my eyes followed hers, and I was in awe of the sight laid out before us. The stars were perfectly illuminated in the sky, and Raye began to point to various constellations and tell me the story of each one. I was fully engrossed in every word she spoke; I felt like a little girl in a planetarium. It was glorious and majestic, and I was pretty sure that even though the stars emitted an intense glow, their brightness was being absorbed in my skin and I was beaming radiant light. She kissed me again, and I knew I would never forget this night for as long as I lived.

The next day when I checked my e-mail, I had an e-card from Raye that had one red rose and said, "Juliet, I'd do the stars with you anytime." It was a line from an Indigo Girls song, "Romeo and Juliet." I was so in love at this point that my smile was plastered on my face permanently.

We spent as much time together after that night as we could—studying, going to dinner, and meeting up on campus for a quick coffee before class. I knew the night would come when we would make love, and I couldn't wait to be with her in that way. After all, it would be my true first time; I discounted the drunken encounters in my past.

One night as we sat in her dorm room on campus, I was at her desk trying to read a textbook as she lay against a large beanbag under her bunk bed. The bunk bed was constructed to have only the top bunk available, since she was a resident assistant in the dorm and had a room to herself. She gestured for me to join her, and my heart stopped—I knew this was it. I went to her and she gently guided me through a beautiful and poetic sexual experience. I had no worries as I navigated her body and held her in me and around me. It was the most natural feeling I had ever experienced to take her in and taste her and let her open me to her. I felt love and passion that I never knew were inside me. I felt safe and comforted. I felt true love for the first time while having sex. We tangled up into one another and, as corny as this sounds, became one.

I woke up the next morning in her arms and just smiled down at her as I eagerly dove under the sheets for another round. Hours and many orgasms later, I glided out of her dorm room to the bus stop. I was overjoyed and felt the sticky sweetness of her all over me. I carried her smell with me all day, and when she rose to meet my nose, it would totally throw my balance off, and I would become giddy with ecstasy. It truly felt like the first time, ever. Even though I'd had such a troubled and vast sexual history—I had never had anything like this.

33

No Means No Sharing

AFTER FINALLY HAVING MY FIRST LESBIAN SEXUAL experience, I felt even more emboldened in my newfound identity. It fit and it felt right. I called Rose and asked her to meet me for coffee. I wanted to share this with someone and my sponsor felt like the right person, even though she had been less than supportive regarding these issues. I must have been beaming so much when I danced into the coffee shop and sat down in front of her, because the look on her face was all scrunched up as though squinting from the sun. I realized quickly that she was not going to want to hear about my night. I decided that instead she and I would have the confrontation I had been avoiding. I said a quiet prayer, set aside my fears, and opened my mouth. I told her that I was going to start looking for a new sponsor and that she just wasn't meeting my emotional needs anymore. I tried to explain that it wasn't personal, that it was me, not her, and that we were growing apart. She wasn't happy, but she understood. After all, every time I would call her to dump my heart out about Raye, she seemed indignant rather than unconditional and supportive—the characteristics that I had grown to rely upon and needed in a sponsor. She just kept rolling out her usual rhetoric, but there was no real connection there anymore. She said she understood, and we would remain friends.

I left the coffee shop feeling like I had just gone through a breakup, and I guess in a way I had. I was sad about hurting Rose's feelings, but also felt good about myself. I was getting better at vocalizing my desires and putting my emotional needs first. I had no idea that this was about to become a skill I would continue to practice.

As the days and weeks passed, Raye and I continued to spend all of our time together, and I loved every second we spent together. I started to notice that she was growing a little distant, and she kept getting interrupted by phone calls from someone while we were together. I didn't really think much of it until one night about a month into our relationship when she came by my apartment. We were supposed to study together, which usually meant we would open our books and pretend to read for about thirty minutes, and then one of us would peek up from behind our books and catch the other doing the same, and before we knew it we were studying each other under the covers. But on this night when she walked up my steps with her usual book bag casually slung across her chest, there was something different in her body language—as if the book bag wasn't the only heavy thing she was carrying. She didn't make a move to sit or take her bag or coat off. She was stiff and seemed to have news that she didn't want to share.

She began to tell me about an older woman whom she had known all her life and they had always been friends, but that she had always known there were feelings there that she wanted to explore, blah blah blah… and before I knew it, I was being dumped—sort of. Instead of breaking up with me, she made me quite the indecent proposal. She wanted me to keep dating her while she explored her feelings with this other woman. She was all innocent eyes and sincerity when she told me that she didn't want to lose me, but also had to see if there was something with this other person.

I couldn't believe this was happening, and instead of crying I just laughed, even though my heart was heading straight into my shoes. In the midst of the ache, I felt a clarity and confidence I had never possessed before. She looked confused. I smiled and stated that I deserved more than that, and if she couldn't give me all of her, then I would rather have nothing. I had heard about these "open relationships" that seemed to be popular around campus, and I knew that I could never exist in one. I was a one-person kind of gal, and while I might share my seat on the bus, I wasn't about to share my bed with more than one person. She looked down at her feet for a while as she shuffled her weight from one foot to the other. "I'm really sorry, Jen. I really do love what we have together. I just know I have to see what could be with her." She seemed all tortured and genuinely upset, and I knew she really believed what she was saying. Raye was nothing but brutally honest. Then her beautiful eyes met mine, and I thought my heart would split in two. I held my ground strongly as she turned on her heel and left my house.

I stood there for a long time looking down the steps, feeling her absence and smelling her lingering scent. I had an odd mixture of emotions running through my body. I knew I loved her and that I wanted nothing more than to be with her, but for the first time in my life, I loved me more. I could easily have said, "Go ahead. See if there is anything with that other woman. I'll be here waiting." And in my past relationships, I was always the type to put the other person first at the painful expense of myself and my needs and feelings. Recovery taught me that I was worth more than that, and I was beginning to believe it. I had integrity and a sense of purpose. I had gotten through so much in my life; I had truly felt and dealt with my emotions. I was strong, and once again I knew I would be okay. I discovered that as much as I wanted her, I didn't need her. I also knew that this experience was happening for a reason, and that whatever pain it might bring would lead me to something better.

During my time in recovery, I began realizing that every time I was in emotional pain, it meant I was actually dealing with something and emotionally or spiritually growing. Each time, I came out on the other side of that pain with clearer insights and feeling stronger than ever before. This would be no exception; I knew there was a lesson in this somewhere.

And while I did cry myself to sleep that night, I woke up feeling the firmness under my feet and walked into the bathroom to start a new day with the knowledge that I was and would be totally fine. Sure, it was hard, and my heart broke like it never had before. Over the next days, weeks, and months, everything reminded me of her—songs, campus, friends. I cried often, the song of the broken-hearted. I spoke her name to anyone who would listen, an act I am sure was growing boring with my sisters in the sorority. But I managed. I got through it.

34

THE GIFT OF MAGI

AFTER RAYE AND I BROKE UP, I WENT TO MY USUAL
home group meeting that night. A home group is a meeting you make
a commitment to attend every week, and you become active in ways
like chairing the meetings and holding a leadership position, such as
treasurer. Twelve-step groups aren't organized in a real formal sense,
but they must have some form of structure to exist. This was a good
meeting for me because Lynn rarely went to it, so it was a safe place for
me to make a weekly commitment to, and it was right next to campus
so I could walk to it quickly. On this particular night I had a lot to
share, and was so grateful to walk into a room of warm and inviting
hellos and hugs. They immediately made me feel better. I was loved and
I was able to show unconditional love in return, which was huge for me.

At this particular meeting, a woman came into the room whom
I had never seen before. I was immediately drawn to her. She was

stunning and had model-type looks—very tall and thin with shoulder-length, dark brown hair and Brooke Shields-like eyebrows. She was gorgeous, and it wasn't every day that women like this walked into the rooms of recovery. She stood out. As we went around the room and shared, I spoke of my heartache. I spilled my guts and found myself crying as I shared. It was so nice to make eye contact as I spoke with other people who I knew understood what I was feeling. To see people shaking their heads in agreement and acknowledgment made me feel so incredibly understood and not alone. I felt so safe in meetings that I often cried openly, because I knew I could wear my pain on my sleeve and the people in my meetings would hand me a tissue and offer me a supportive hug. I then began rambling on about how I really needed a job to take my mind off things and to make some money. I didn't want a ton of responsibility because I was very busy with school and my activities, but I wanted something that would earn me some extra cash.

After I spoke, the new woman, whose name was Magi, spoke of how she was new to the area but not to recovery; in fact, she had a significant amount of clean time. She talked about how much she could relate to what I was saying because she was going through a similar situation. As I listened to her speak, I felt connected to her instantly. She then spoke of her two small children whom she needed help with, as she had just moved to town on her own. We both just looked at each other and smiled, knowing we had just found what we were looking for and more. I approached her after the meeting and introduced myself. We chitchatted, and then I asked her if I could help with her children and we exchanged phone numbers. We formed a wonderful friendship, and I began babysitting her children a couple of times a week while she ran a children's clothing store in town. It was a great situation, and I immediately fell in love with her two beautiful little girls, who were two and five years old.

After a couple weeks of getting to know one another and my watching her children, it became abundantly clear that Magi and I had so much in common. She was born and raised in Allentown and did a good deal of her using there before she moved to New York City to model. Our histories were eerily similar. I felt like she was me, only ten years older. We clicked, and I found myself calling her with my woes about Raye and other life-related stuff. She gave great advice.

One day it hit me that she was really the best sponsor I had—even though she wasn't my sponsor. I asked Magi to be my sponsor that day, and she accepted. It was a perfect fit, and I finally felt like I had a kindred spirit in the program. She just got me, but we were so alike that she was also really good at calling me on my shit. Magi was and still is definitely a soul mate of mine, and I was so grateful that she and her children were brought into my life in that moment. We needed each other in different ways. I helped her get her new life in State College on track by being her first friend and helping with the kids, and she gave me an incredibly blissful distraction from my heartache in the form of her two girls. I loved every second I spent with them. They brought out the little kid in me, and we played every week. It was such a wondrous feeling to let myself be totally free and childlike with them. We had a blast together and really grew to love one another. They became a family for me, and Magi became not just a sponsor but a best friend and more. She was the sister I never had but always dreamt of.

35

SOCIOLOGY LESSONS

IN 2000, I BECAME MORE ACTIVE ON CAMPUS IN THE gay community. I joined the sorority, and at Dr. Rankin's suggestion, I also joined a couple of other gay groups that were active on campus. Pledging the sorority was amazing, even though it meant I would see Raye quite often. Joining something with all its traditions and activities made me feel a part of something that was unique, and it made me feel bonded to these women. When I saw Raye, my stomach did flip-flops and my heart ached. I managed to get through it all by diving head-on into pledging activities, which meant spending a lot of time with my pledge class and getting to know the other sisters. I had to set up a one-on-one meeting with each sister, and as a pledge class we had to put on socials for the sorority so we could all get to know one another. I was getting involved in activist work with the organizations Dr. Rankin hooked me up with and began getting involved in rallies, pride events, and other social activities on campus for the gay community. I was also babysitting the girls often, so there was little time to think about Raye.

I put my energy into learning as much as I could in school and focusing on my recovery work. I read a lot of recovery books when I wasn't reading for school. I loved to read, and enjoyed reading stories of other people in recovery—it helped keep things in perspective for me. I was so busy on campus and found myself spending more and more time there, so I decided to see if there were any meetings on campus. It made sense to me that there would be. I called the health building and inquired about it, but they informed me that at the time there were no recovery meetings on campus. I didn't let that stop me; I decided to start my own. I figured if I couldn't get to a meeting as often as I wanted to, then I would bring the meeting to me. I went to the student union office and found out what I needed to do. I submitted a request to reserve a room once a week at noon for a twelve-step meeting. I collected all the literature I needed for the meetings and brought in my own books to use. My request was accepted, and I was ecstatic! I made flyers and hung them all over campus, as well as listing the meeting in the college newspaper and on all the community events web pages. I was so excited that now I had a meeting to attend right on campus each week between classes. The meetings were never packed, but we always had a good mix of staff, faculty, and students attending. Many of the faculty and staff thanked me, saying that there had never been a recovery meeting on campus before and that it was so nice to be able to take their lunches and come to a meeting during work.

I began taking lots of sociology courses and was flabbergasted by the number of things I didn't learn growing up and how incredibly limited and inaccurate my sources of information were. I learned of things like racism, oppression, and the Holocaust, to name just a few— events and realizations that were not a part of my vernacular growing up. I realized my father was racist and had taught me to be racist, even though he would never agree with that statement.

When I was five years old, I would go to my brothers' baseball games with them. I didn't particularly like the games, so I would often gather with other younger siblings and play with them. There was a cemetery right next to one field, and I would play there with a boy, Mike, whom I grew very fond of and who also happened to be the only black boy at the game. His older brother played baseball, and he and I would play together during games.

One day while we were running through the cemetery, Mike pushed me and I fell into a headstone. It threw me off a bit, but I wasn't really hurt in any physical way. But what came out of my mouth would hurt this boy in a very deep, emotional way. I casually called him a "nigger." He looked like I had slapped him across the face, and I stood there confused in his wake as he began to cry and took off running toward his parents. I wasn't quite sure what had happened, but I had a feeling that I was in big trouble. I walked slowly back toward the field, and as I looked up from my feet, my eyes met a commotion as his father approached my father. The look on my dad's face as he saw me approach confirmed my feeling that I was in trouble. I glanced over at Mike, who was being comforted by his mother. She had a pained, proud look on her face as she comforted her son. My father grabbed me by the arm and walked me over to Mike and made me apologize to him and his family. I did as I was told, and as the apology fell out of my mouth, so did the tears from my eyes. My father scolded me, saying in a loud voice, "You are grounded, young lady."

I was incredibly puzzled—confused that a word I heard flow freely around the confines of my own home from my own parents was so different in the light of day around others. I had heard my parents say this word a bazillion times in our home when referring to black people. I never knew what it meant or that it would cause the pain on a face the way it did on Mike's when he looked up at me. I didn't understand how my father could be so visibly angry at me for something he taught me. I kept it all inside and accepted my consequences.

My father ranted the whole way home about how embarrassed he was, but never really mentioned that what I said was wrong. He and my mother were upset about how it made them look and what people thought. Turns out I wasn't grounded or anything when we got home, which left me more baffled. I didn't understand if the word was wrong or if directing it at a person was wrong. I didn't ask, because I never really questioned anything my parents told me when I was young.

Years later, while sitting in Dr. Richards's sociology class learning about oppression and racism, the memory of that incident flooded my mind and hit me in the stomach like a ton of bricks. That was the day I learned what true hypocrisy was, and at that tender age I couldn't tell you what that word was, but I felt it in every fiber of my being. I felt dirty with it. I sat in class feeling the shame of it all, and the guilt that began to creep into my soul that day made me stiff. I wasn't a hateful person, this I knew; I was raised to believe certain things were one way, and that was all I knew. I was now learning they weren't that way at all. It was overwhelming and invigorating at the same time. There is incredible truth in the saying "ignorance is bliss," for you cannot be upset about something you know nothing of. You cannot change something until you own it to be true, until you acknowledge that it actually exists—much like I couldn't change my addiction until I was ready to admit it was a problem. Denial is a very real concept.

I felt like I was uncovering truths that affected my life in a deep, meaningful way, and when I would go home to visit with my parents, I felt the need to pour out my revelations onto their kitchen table for them to examine. My father was incredibly critical of this, and the more I learned about the welfare of our nation and our social system and its flaws and discrimination, the degradation of people and the injustices that were occurring and had occurred all around the world, the more my father came to resent my education. We began arguing about politics in a fierce way. I would come home armed with this information and carry a youthful resentment toward him for not sharing this with me when I was young. I would take aim and fire my rhetoric in his direction and await his response, and no matter what he came back with, I had my racket ready to bounce my opinion back at him.

We would go back and forth for hours like this, one insult flung after another, a parental struggle of wits and values flung out over the dinner table night after night, with my unwilling stepmother playing referee. The conversations would always end with my father calling me a communist and throwing me out of the country for daring to be so un-American by challenging his views. I felt that I was more American than I had ever been in my life. I felt that finally I was engaging in a process that I had never realized even existed. I held a responsibility for the education I was receiving in the palm of my hand with dignity and purpose.

It was as though I had a new job, and now that I knew that life was one way and not the way I was taught, I was making it my goal in life to create change. To influence others, to expound on the injustices, I leaned upon every ear that would listen. To say I was dogmatic is an understatement! But having walked through so much of life totally ignorant to all that surrounded me, I felt it was my duty to make up for lost time. I had been shielded and had shielded myself for too long, encapsulated by my own ignorance. I had been like a small child, believing I was the only one in the world with needs and desires. I had been childishly selfish in my isolation from the day-to-day struggles of anyone other than myself. Recovery helped me realize how big the world was and that, as much as I thought it did, it did not revolve around me.

36

COMING OUT IN SOBS

I DECIDED IT WAS TIME TO COME OUT TO MY PARENTS
once and for all. I was beginning to understand the oppression of gay
people in our culture, and I knew that I could no longer be a part
of it. By not coming out to everyone in my life, I was an active part
of the problem. I chose to do this during Easter break, since I was
home visiting my parents at the time. Most people, organizations, and
counselors will tell you to avoid holidays for such revelations, but I was
in college and it wasn't like I had a ton of opportunities to tell them. I
had felt so deceptive, like I was living a big lie, and with my recovering
principles governing my new life, it just didn't jibe with how I wanted
to live my life. Honesty was now the cornerstone of my existence. How
could I look them in the eyes when I knew I was hiding such a huge
part of who I was? My phone calls to them began to get more strained,
because I couldn't really tell them what I was doing at school. I couldn't

talk to them about the fact that I had fallen head over heels and had my heart broken. It felt dishonest and shady, and that wasn't who I was anymore.

In doing my step work, I had already made my amends with them. It was a very powerful moment for us, even though my parents' attempts to be codependent kept getting us off track. They knew the steps, so they knew at some point it was coming, and on the day I went to them to make my amends for all the things I had done, they did everything they could to make it okay. They couldn't stand to see me emotional, so they tried to interrupt about a dozen times by saying, "We know, Jennifer, and it's okay." But I pushed on and continued to get everything out that I needed to say. After all, amends aren't so much for the other person as they are for us. It is a major part of my emotional healing in recovery that I own up to all the shit I did in the past, and that means apologizing for hurting people. It makes sense, really—how can you move forward into a clean and healthy life if you have wreckage from your past hanging over your head? I embraced my amends because I didn't want to fear bumping into someone from my past whom I might have harmed in some way and having to avoid them or just having that horrible feeling in the pit of my stomach. Recovery was all about keeping my side of the street clean, and that meant taking out a whole lot of old and stinky trash.

So here I was, about to take another huge step in my recovery, and this one wasn't covered in any of the literature that I'd read.

I was scared because I had heard horror stories of those who had gone home and come out to their parents, only to find themselves disowned and homeless or pulled out of college altogether and placed immediately into therapy. I figured since I was already in therapy, that was not too likely to happen, but I was still concerned about how my parents would react. They had never done anything but love me unconditionally throughout the years, and even in those moments that my father was throwing me out of the country for my new beliefs, he still hugged me and told me he loved me before bed.

I borrowed a friend's car and drove home for the weekend. During the entire drive home I practiced my speech in the rearview mirror, going over and over what I would say and how I would say it. I had butterflies in my stomach and had to stop multiple times on the road because I was sick to my stomach. I had told my sponsor what I was doing that weekend, and she was on call for me just in case I needed her. I called her multiple times on my drive down, going over every possible scenario that could occur. What if they disowned me? What if they hated me? What if they made me leave? I poured all of my fears into the receiver of my cell phone, and Magi eased each one as I threw it at her. She assured me that no matter what, my parents would love me, and that no matter what their initial reaction might be, I would be okay. She was wonderful, and I was so incredibly grateful to have her on the other end of the phone.

I sat my stepmother and father down at the kitchen table. I pulled up all the strength I could find, opened my mouth to tell them, and—nothing came out but a burst of sobs. I slobbered all over the table as emotions washed over me and spilled onto my very concerned and confused parents. My father's eyes immediately became red and sullen as he looked right at me and asked me what was wrong. I could tell he was bracing himself for the worst news possible. After all, nothing would surprise this man after what he had been through with me. I didn't want to prolong his pain by not responding, so I took in what felt like all the air in the room, and when it reached my throat, I exhaled it back into the room with the words "I'm gay." And I sat there, deflated and waiting... .

My parents' postures straightened up as they quickly exchanged glances of what seemed to be relief. My father let out a deep belly laugh and said, "Oh, thank God. I thought you were pregnant." With that, I joined him in his laughter as I eyed my mother, who laughed with us, but I noticed it was forced and there was a cloudiness of unease behind her eyes that came through her smile. They didn't have any questions. They just went back about their business in the kitchen to prepare for dinner, and I retreated to my bedroom. It was all surreal, and I was thrilled that they weren't horrified or sad, even though I knew my stepmother's eyes exposed something that I would have to deal with some other time. But on that day, I just wanted to relish the knowledge that I was finally free, living my life with 100 percent honesty, and that was enough.

I went back to college feeling totally unencumbered and ready to explore everything I could about myself and the world. That was really the beauty of college—all the self-examination and exploration was invigorating. Every day was an adventure. More and more, I began to strip away all the things that I had thought made up my personality; the girly clothes, the heavy makeup were gone. The sense of self I was gathering was strengthening almost every day. It no longer seemed important or vital for me to hide my face under makeup. I grew to love my face, and when I would walk out of my house fresh-faced with not a bit of makeup on, I felt free and beautiful. I still had long hair, which at the time I was dyeing a deep red. I had dyed my hair a million times in my life; just like I changed my clothes and makeup, my hair always followed suit. But it had started to itch as of late and didn't feel right anymore. I couldn't even have told you what my natural hair color was if you paid me, because I had been covering it up for years.

One day, while at the mall with some of my new sorority sisters, I decided to cut it off. Almost all my friends now, who were of course gay or bisexual, had super-short hair. It was "the look." I decided I was ready to free myself from my long hair and join them. I sat in the chair as the woman looked at my beautifully long and thick hair and asked me skeptically if I was sure. I nodded yes, and she cut my hair to about three inches in length. I walked out of the mall feeling incredibly light but a little uncertain of my new hair. That night I went to a party with all my sorority sisters, and I knew Raye was going to be there. It had been months since we'd been together. I was nervous about what she would think of my new hair. As I walked into the party, all eyes were on me and everyone kept gushing the way people do when a person makes a drastic change in their appearance. Raye wasn't there yet, and my self-confidence built as people kept telling me how cool my hair looked and how they were astonished at what I'd done. Then Raye walked in, hand in hand with some new woman she was dating. Apparently she had broken up with the woman she left me for and was already on to some other heavy-set, older woman. I couldn't believe she was with someone else, and just like that, my self-confidence took a header. I couldn't stand being in the same room with her as she laughed and hung on this woman. I couldn't breathe, and I excused myself to go to the bathroom upstairs. While I sat on the toilet lid attempting to gather myself, Shannon, whose house I was in, came in to comfort me. She was a great friend and always ready with a totally inappropriate joke to cheer me up, and it started to work. I was feeling a little bit better and stood up to fix my face, and I saw myself in the mirror. My hair was a mess because I wasn't quite sure how to style my new short 'do—my hair was so thick that it just kind of looked like an afro. My eye caught sight of a hair clipper sitting on the edge of the bathroom sink. Shannon had super-short hair and apparently must have trimmed her own. I looked up at her and said, "Cut it all off."

She just looked at me like I was nuts, and with a half-assed smile, blew me off, saying, "Girl, you're crazy." I looked at her with all the seriousness I could manage and said, "I'm serious; it looks terrible and doesn't feel right. Cut it off." She grew serious and looked me right in the eye and said, "Are you sure?" "Yes," I said. Without another word I sat on the toilet lid, and she began shearing off the three inches that was left of my hair. While we were doing this, another one of my friends came in and shouted, "Holy shit, Storm, what are you doing?" Shannon and I laughed, and my other friend grabbed a pair of scissors and helped her cut my hair. Before I knew it I was surrounded by a bunch of my sorority sisters, who began taking turns cutting my hair off. We were all laughing hysterically, and at one point Raye came up to see what all the commotion was about. She looked at me, but I couldn't meet her gaze, and her mouth dropped when she saw what was going on. "Jen, what are you doing?" she asked in amazement. Without looking at her, I just shrugged and said coldly, "I needed a change." Everyone in the room was quiet. They all knew about Raye and me and how hurt I was. Raye walked out of the bathroom, and we resumed our hair-cutting party. After every last strand had fallen to the floor, I just sat there staring at it all under and around my feet. I asked everyone to leave, and I stood up, closed the door, and turned to see in the mirror what I had just done. I saw myself, but totally different. For the first time—I saw me. I was bare, no makeup, no hair, standing there in a white T-shirt. I ran my hand over my newly bald head and just smiled. My head was actually a pretty decent shape. Deep down, I felt something rise in my soul—it was confidence. My deep blue eyes stared back at me from the mirror, and for the first time in my life I really recognized the woman looking back. There was nothing left to hide beneath, no hair to let fall over my eyes to shield me from what I didn't want to see, no makeup to plaster over an expression I didn't want the world to see. Just me. My skin and my flesh laid bare. I was gorgeous, and I felt it. I was free. I had never felt so light in all of my life. I was truly a clean slate. I walked out of that bathroom with such a newfound assurance that I didn't even notice Raye as I left the party. I was a new woman.

37

TOKEN DYKE

BY THE SPRING OF 2000, EVERYTHING WAS FALLING
into place in my life. I was doing well in college, had a great sponsor,
and had a wonderful group of new friends whom I loved spending
time with. I was still making several meetings a week, including the
one I had started on campus, and since I had completed my Twelve
Steps, I sought out a way to carry my message to those who were sick
and suffering with addiction. I knew I had a powerful message of
hope to share as a young person, and was ready to start taking that
message outside the rooms of recovery. I contacted the local drug and
alcohol office in State College to see if there was any way I could be of
assistance. They hooked me up with the drug- and alcohol-awareness
classes that many first- and second-time offenders were mandated to
take. I began going to those classes on a monthly basis and sharing my
story with them. It was an incredible way to give back, and I found
immense gratification in explaining to people where I came from and

how I got to be where I was now. I also began sponsoring some young women in the program, another wonderful opportunity for me to give back. It also helped keep me and my recovery in check at all times. I found sponsorship to be not only a great way to guide other people through the process, but a wonderful way for me to continue my own focus on recovery while working the steps again with them.

I was heavily involved on campus in every organization I could find that had a queer element. I was also a teaching assistant in my sociology class on race and ethnic relations. Twice a week, I would run a small group where we dissected the issues of race, sexuality, ethnicity, and religion. It forced us to stretch the reality that each of us came to college with. Some people who had never in their lives seen a gay person or black person were finding themselves intermixed in a multicultural environment and it caused great tension, confusion, fear, and ignorance. My professor, Dr. Sam Richards, taught the course, and his wife, Dr. Laurie Mulvey, mentored all the teaching assistants and helped usher us through this complex journey in the hope of creating acceptance and understanding of one another through these breakout sessions in our sociology class. I was honored to have been chosen as one of their teaching assistants. It was an honor bestowed upon a large handful of students each semester who both Sam and Laurie felt not only embodied some of the multiculturalism they sought to teach, but in whom they had seen something deeper. I was beyond flattered when they asked me. I was clearly the token dyke, and I was totally comfortable with that acknowledgment. It had truly become my primary identity.

After I'd shaved off all my hair, I kept it super-short. I wore my lesbian identity on my sleeve—literally. My backpacks were littered with buttons that screamed such slogans as "I'm here. I'm queer. Get used to it."

By this time I had become well known on campus as what was jokingly referred to as the BLOC: the Big Lesbian On Campus. This was a title that went to one lesbian who really stood out on the campus and took charge of the community by getting involved in as many queer leadership positions as possible. When I first came to school, my sorority sister Ann, who was a senior, held the title. Since Ann had graduated, the title had been handed down to me. This I accepted with great pride. I found that I was a natural-born leader. I was planning events, organizing protests, writing letters to the editor, and appearing in the college newspaper almost weekly as the gay spokesperson for the student body. I was on speed-dial with the newspaper's reporting staff. Anytime they had a question about anything gay, they called me. I cannot tell you how many times my picture was on the front of the newspaper holding a rainbow flag or protest sign, or speaking at a rally. From time to time I was on the local news when their reporters came on campus to cover our events. I was at home in this role and found myself totally engrossed in being gay.

As I was learning in my sociology and psychology classes, this was common in many cultures when a person begins to self-identify with their roots, whether that is their racial background, ethnicity, religious affiliation, or sexuality. I learned in college that when a person first identifies with these things deeply, they go through certain developmental phases, such as the identity or immersion phase. I was in what the gay community refers to as my "pride phase," when one identifies solely with the group and then becomes totally immersed in that culture, making sure that everyone around them is aware of their affiliation. I wore my queerness like a badge of honor. I aligned it with how I immersed myself in the program of recovery when I first got clean and sober. My entire world revolved around recovery, and while it was still a very large part of my life on a daily basis, my recovery was enabling me to branch out in other ways. I was in my third year of recovery, and I carried my two-year medallion with me wherever I went, always serving as a reminder of where I came from and how far I had come.

I also noticed that while I received a great deal of admiration and acceptance from my peers, my reality in the world was different with my newfound identity. People looked at me oddly when I walked down the street. I was followed in stores by clerks who would have usually bent over backwards to help me. Now they eyed me suspiciously, like I was going to steal something. I began to fully understand what it meant to be a minority, to be looked upon as an outsider. It was easier being gay when I still looked "straight" with my makeup and long hair. I could still blend easily into both worlds without being detected. But now, with my new looks, it was abundantly clear what and who I was to the world. With my ultrashort haircut and outwardly gay appearance, it wasn't out of place for me to be walking on campus and hear the word "dyke" muttered in disgust by another student walking by. Worse, in the evenings when students were a bit more emboldened by their extracurricular drinking activities, it wasn't uncommon to have a group of guys scream "fucking queers" or "fucking dykes" at a group of us as we walked on campus. It made my blood boil and also made me very sad inside that people who didn't even know me would have such hatred for me based solely on my appearance.

Even though I had a great deal of pride in who I was now and felt firmly positioned in my own life the way I knew I was supposed to be, it still hurt at times to feel the hate that sometimes surrounded me. I was in central Pennsylvania, and even though I was attending an institution of higher learning, I was living in what most Pennsylvanians would jokingly refer to as the "Alabama" part of the state. Pittsburgh is at one end and Philadelphia at the other—both major metropolitan areas with mostly Democratic views—and then you have "Alabama" running though the middle of the state. We are a swing state in most elections because of this eclectic makeup. Central Pennsylvania is mostly rural and vastly conservative, home to farmers, hunters, working-class folks who tend to the Republican side, and what I would soon find—hate groups. Pennsylvania was home to many nationally affiliated, organized hate groups. Little did I realize I would soon become acquainted with one in particular. It made me stronger in my resolve to change beliefs and behaviors of others. It just made me work harder at the events I was planning, as I had a strong purpose behind each and every action.

38

QUEER PROM

ONE EVENT IN WHICH I WAS HEAVILY ENGROSSED was the planning of the first-ever Penn State Queer Prom. It was to be our end-of-the-year main event for 2000. I wanted to provide an experience for the queer kids on campus that they were never able to have in high school. Most queer young people went to prom either with someone of the opposite gender or not at all. It is a rite of passage that is often taken away from queer people, or at the very least, is not experienced fully like it is for most students.

I had never had so many close friends in all of my life as I did during my time in State College, including three amazing gay guy friends who were helping me plan the prom. As we got ready for the first prom, I was giddy with excitement. I had spent countless hours examining every detail of this event so it would be fabulous. At the time, I was casually dating Ann, but everyone knew my heart still belonged to Raye, so my efforts with Ann were futile at best. I had a few hot encounters with other women, but none of them felt right. Since I was all about being true to myself, I didn't last long in any dating or relationship scenarios. I had heard that Raye had broken up with her latest, and she and I were speaking every now and then. Our attraction had never gone away; even when she was dating other women, we would talk or see each other at a party and wind up making out all night in the corner or even, one particular night, in a kitchen sink. But she had still been involved with the other person, and I wasn't going to push her until she was ready. I still thought deep down that we would wind up together; I felt it was our destiny.

It turns out I was right. She ended up showing up at the prom dateless and swept me off my feet as we danced all night. Ann and I were not on any official type of date that night, so Raye and I were free to spend the evening together. That night she came to my apartment as I slept and threw stones at my window until I woke to find her standing outside with a rose and a smile. I let her back into my apartment, my bedroom, and my heart that night, and she never left. We became an official couple, and this time it was for good.

So my life was perfect, as it seemed. I had a ton of wonderful friends, school was going well, I was totally in love with an amazing woman, and my parents seemed to be okay with everything. I began bringing Raye around, and even though they were timid, they were tolerant. My stepmother had a hard time at first. I truly think they both thought my venture into the gay world was a college phase, but once I brought Raye home and had an "official girlfriend," it began to sink in to them that this was no phase. They began to fall in love with Raye as much as I did—it was pretty hard not to love her. Getting to know my family was eye-opening for her. She came from a religious family that really lived the American dream. There was no trauma in her history, and she struggled to understand the family I came from. She never judged us; she accepted my dysfunctional family unconditionally, and I think it was that unconditional spirit and love that ended up bonding her and my stepmother so well. They were both female outsiders brought into this insanity of a family by people they couldn't help but love. Raye and my stepmother shared that commonality and it brought them together, and out of that, my stepmother's acceptance of our love came freely.

Raye and I dated all through our junior year, and I stayed extremely active on campus. I was committed to the community and truly came into my own as an activist. I continued to be the "go-to" person for media and everyone else on campus when it came to gay issues, and I became the president of the sorority.

This latest role didn't go over as well as I would have hoped. I quickly learned that when you become a leader in a community, it can be a very lonely place to be. Once you are seen as a person of authority, people tend to resent you a bit. It was a lesson in leadership that was challenging for me, and Dr. Rankin really mentored me through that process. It was one she had come to know all too well, being a leader on campus herself.

My sorority sisters treated me differently as I tried to steer us away from the party scene and more into community service. I cannot blame them in hindsight; we clearly had different priorities. Even though I was okay around the party scene because they were respectful of my recovery, I took the sorority in a direction they weren't all thrilled with.

I was so compelled and committed to trying to change beliefs and attitudes and make a difference on campus that sometimes I forgot that some people just wanted to have fun. That is where my difference in age and my recovery were glaringly clear. I saw these strong, beautiful, and intelligent women within the group as agents of change, just as I was, and in many ways they just weren't there yet in their own lives. They were still into hooking up and hanging out, while I was on a mission to change the world.

I felt we were at a critical mass. Matthew Shepard, a gay student in Wyoming, had been murdered a few years earlier in 1998. As a result, outrage was being expressed across the nation about the way gay people were treated in society. For the first time nationally, people took notice of the hatred that was expressed against gay people. I think it was because Matthew was a white, male college student with an affluent family. His image hit home with many families in that "Oh my goodness, he could be anyone's son" kind of way. I just wanted to capitalize on that, to try to educate people about who we were, to try to somehow infuse acceptance into an intolerant rural community. I felt such an internal compulsion to make a difference on campus, because for me and for so many of us, it was a life-or-death situation at times. I often found myself in Dr. Rankin's office in tears of frustration and conflict. She guided me through it all and helped me realize that I was a little different from the average college student.

It was so hard for me to balance being a recovery person, with all my grown-up history and experience under my belt, with this new, young college student that I had become. Sometimes I felt like I totally fit in, and other times I felt like I was so alone that no one in the world understood my plight. People in the rooms understood, and I relied heavily upon their understanding and guidance, but once I would step out of a meeting and back onto campus—it was once again another world. While I was happy and felt blessed to have so many friends, there was still always the underlying knowledge that I was different. I couldn't just tune out the world around me as others were able to do so freely. Recovery had awakened me, and now that I was aware of what was going on around me, I felt a strong sense of purpose. I was becoming an activist, and that isn't always a popular role.

39

SOMETHING IN THE WATER

ONE NIGHT I GOT A CALL FROM MY PARENTS TELLING me that Brian had been arrested and was in jail. He and my brother Jimmy were still deeply struggling with addiction. Jimmy had tried rehab a couple of times and had lived in a halfway house for a time where he was doing very well, but then he would have a slip and it would be back to the usual.

This time Brian had gotten into a fight with a police officer and wound up in jail. My parents told me they were not going to bail him out. I was so proud of them, because they had been such enablers to all of us as we each struggled with addiction. Like so many parents of addicts, they wanted nothing more than a good life for their children and they made countless sacrifices both financially and emotionally to ensure our safety. But unfortunately they never really could secure our recovery or safety—just as no parent can. It is a futile effort when dealing with an addicted child.

My father used duct tape in an attempt to fix me. When I used to drink and black out—which was more often than I care to recall—I wasn't the best driver. I drank, and I drove, and I bounced off things all over town including utility poles, other vehicles, sidewalks, walls—you name it—if it happened to cross the path of my vehicle while I was intoxicated and driving, I hit it. I am not proud of this; it was simply the reality of my life and my addiction at the time. I would often awaken from a night of heavy drinking and have a fog of emptiness in my head where the memories of the last evening should have been. I would find my father fixing my car with, of course, duct tape. Whether it be a smashed light or my fender half hanging down from hitting a riser on the road, he would be there quietly, lovingly duct-taping the parts back together.

I would always act as if I had no idea what happened, which in essence was the truth; I rarely had any recollection of the prior evening's events, and in the rare case when I did remember bouncing off something, I never admitted it to my father. I would just dismissively say, "Oh, someone must have hit me in the parking lot," and thank him for fixing the damage for me while never making eye contact with him.

I know he knew that I was lying. I know he taped my vehicle because he loved me and wanted to protect me, and also because he felt unable to help me in any other way. My disease was full-blown and directly in his face, and there was nothing he could do to stop me from getting behind the wheel on any given night and drinking and driving. It was his way of trying to put me back together, part by part, piece of tape by piece of tape. He fixed my vehicle in the absence of his ability to fix me. It was the one thing he felt he had some type of control over.

My parents had gone to twelve-step meetings with me and really began to grasp the program of recovery and their role in it. They began to learn about their codependency and enabling behaviors. It was a large step for them to not bail Brian out of jail, and I knew it was one that kept them both up at night, riddled with guilt. But sometimes the healthy choices that we must make for those we love hurt us the most. Brian stayed in jail for a couple of weeks, and upon his release when he called my parents for a ride home, they didn't answer the phone. Brian walked home that day. It was several miles to my parents' home, and on that walk he had an awakening. He realized his life was completely unmanageable and he was sick and tired of being sick and tired. By the time he reached my parents' house, his feet were killing him but his heart was a bit lighter. He decided to take everyone's advice and go to rehab. He went to the same rehab I had gone to three years earlier. He did well there, as he admitted freely that he was in fact an addict, and he began rigorously working a program of recovery. After thirty days, he went on to live in a sober living home right outside State College, which thrilled me. He and his other housemates would drive into State College every Saturday morning and attend our meetings. It was amazing to have my brother in the rooms with me, talking about recovery and looking better and healthier each time I saw him. I felt like my prayers had been answered. I was so proud of him that I would beam when he came into a meeting, and I made sure everyone within earshot knew he was my brother—not like you couldn't tell just by looking at us, since we resembled each other so much. It was so nice to have someone from my family in State College.

After the sober living house, Brian moved to State College with another male friend. He attended meetings with me, and we began to build our bond back in a new and exciting way. I had my brother back, and it felt amazing. We began to get to know one another again as people in recovery, and I loved spending time with him and sharing funny stories of our childhood. I had such a tainted view of my childhood as a result of all the trauma and damage that had been done that it was nice to recall the good times with him and know they were real. My parents couldn't have been happier, and even though Jimmy still struggled, they now had two children who they knew were safe and in recovery. They were beginning to think that there was something in the water in State College!

40

Death and Protest

I WAS ONLY ONE YEAR AWAY FROM GRADUATION,
which was scary since Raye and I weren't sure what we wanted to do
after college, and I had everything I had ever wanted: a wonderful
love, a great community, a new education, self-awareness that made
me glow, my brother in recovery and living near me, and a future that
seemed limitless.

Raye had been active in the Special Olympics and got me involved
as well. I began coaching volleyball and softball—two sports I had
no business coaching, really. However, it wasn't about skill with the
Special Olympics, it was about having fun, and I sure had a whole
lot to offer in that area—which was good because most of the young
athletes kicked my butt in both sports. It was about motivating them
and helping them reach a new goal. In many ways I related so much
to the athletes, because I knew what it was like to have to overcome

something and the glory you felt once you reached a goal, no matter how small. I found myself very emotional at times when working with them because I felt so blessed to have the opportunity to do it. It made me feel even more in awe of recovery and its gifts. The best part of it all was what I got from the athletes: they made me see myself in a whole new way. They helped me slow down, set aside my ego, and appreciate the simple joys of life on an even deeper level. It was a humbling experience. Working a program of recovery in my life meant getting out of myself as often as I could and being of service to others.

Raye and I were getting serious and decided to get a house together. Raye was done being a resident assistant and wanted to get out of the dorms, so we started looking and found an adorable rental right behind the house of Joe Paterno, the head football coach at Penn State since 1966. I walked past his humble home every day and couldn't believe someone who was so famous and made so much money lived in such a modest home. I loved our little home, and soon after we moved in we brought home a rat terrier/Jack Russell mix that we named Tanner. He and my cat got along very well, and suddenly Raye and I had a little family. I couldn't imagine life being any better.

And then the world came down around me and everyone else. I was sitting in my anthropology class at 8:45 a.m. on the morning of September 11, 2001, when a couple of minutes later my professor came in to announce that there was some accident at the World Trade Center. He didn't go into details, and as all the students began to pour out of his classroom, I saw a look on his face that disturbed me. I walked briskly to the student union building where my organization's office was, which was only about a minute away from my class. I could feel the energy shift on campus. As I walked, I heard people buzzing with words like "plane" and "New York City," and as I approached the student union building there was a sea of students sitting on the floor in front of the massive flat-screen TV in the center of the building. I saw the image of a smoking World Trade Center, where a plane had apparently crashed into the upper part of the building.

I listened for less than a minute to the commentary and surveyed the crowd around me. Some students were quietly talking on cell phones; most just looked on in confusion, as I did. I gathered myself and rushed to the elevator that went to the third floor where my office was. I felt uneasy, but had no clue what was happening. It was very odd that a commercial jet would hit a building, I thought. As the door opened to the third floor, I stepped out just in time to look up at the TV set that hung right outside my office and see a plane hit the south side of the second tower. I gasped as white, fluffy clouds of smoke emerged from the building, but the plane never did. There was a rush of reporters beginning to talk of "terrorist attack" on TV. I pulled my chair out of my office and sat down to watch the coverage. My whole body was frozen as I watched this massive commercial plane smack into the side of a building and disappear, replayed over and over again. It was haunting, and impossible to look away from. Moments later, there were reports of a plane hitting the Pentagon. A panic rose in me, and I was glued to the TV. I sat in silence, listening to the scrambling reporters try to confirm information coming into the station as they continued to replay the footage of the second plane crash. After about fifteen minutes, a reporter said there were reports that another plane went down in Shanksville, Pennsylvania, and my entire insides went numb. I didn't know where Shanksville was; all I heard was Pennsylvania and all I could think of was my family. I thought I might puke as I ran to the phone in my office and immediately dialed my parents. I reached my stepmother, who was at work. By this time I was sobbing uncontrollably, asking if they were okay and screaming hysterically about this being the next world war. My stepmother was also in tears, and she tried to reassure me that everyone was okay. I spoke to my father. Then I called Raye, who was working at the time as a security officer on campus. She was leaving work and coming over to my office right away. She got there just as the first tower collapsed, and as it did, I collapsed into her arms.

Raye and I held vigil in front of our television, as did the entire nation, for what seemed like days. The images were being played and replayed. It was as though the whole world was on a broken record that no one could fix, and we all kept reliving the trauma over and over again. I just sat, crying. I cried myself to sleep that night and had a fear inside me that I had never known before. Could this be the end of the world? Was it over? Would more things happen? If I closed my eyes and allowed myself to sleep, would I wake up? And if so, what would I awake to? I didn't sleep that night. Instead I just watched the news. I was obsessed with the coverage. I couldn't take my eyes off the TV because I was afraid I would miss something else happening.

Tensions on campus were heating up as acts of hate were being played out everywhere. It started with an Asian female who went missing one night—simply vanished into thin air. Her name was Cindy Song, and many students organized to try to find her, but the University seemed more interested in trying to explain it away. My organization was working closely with the Black Caucus at the time, and the leaders of that organization had been receiving death threats— black football players, and then even the board of trustees started receiving them as well. There were swastikas drawn on dorms outside of a Jewish boy's room. A gay boy was attacked outside his dorm. It seemed like every week something hateful was happening to minority students. Every incident made the paper, and there was energy on campus that was making everyone's skin crawl, except for the apathetic students who weren't affected or simply didn't care or, worse, who were involved. It seems that people just had a license to hate after the attacks. No one was safe, unless of course you were a white male.

With each incident, the threats to student leaders were becoming worse. Notes threatened that the body of a black student would be found. The university, in an attempt to respond, decided to plan a unity march to stop the hate. University officials sent a mass e-mail to the entire student body about the march. The student leaders who had received the death threats felt like it was a poor way to respond to threats being made on lives, which it was. Thousands of people gathered for the march, but instead of having it, the students took it over and demanded that the university president take an actual stand against what was happening by meeting with the students and talking about a much-needed change in culture on campus. The university president refused, so instead of the march hundreds of us went to the student union and held a ten-day sit-in protest, demanding protection as well as more diversity programs at the university.

The threatening letters had spanned about two years. In November 1999, more than sixty students had received racist e-mail messages signed by "The Patriot." Those e-mails were traced to a site about 200 miles from campus. The threatening letters intensified as black student leaders pressed the university to enhance its diversity programs. I joined the black student leaders and, for the first time in Penn State's history, unified the gay organization with the Black Caucus. We became a tight-knit group that worked hard to create much-needed change on campus. I became closer to some of these people than I had to anyone I had ever known in my life. The shared conviction and passion we all had for creating this change brought us together as family.

Sleeping bags and students littered the student union building's floor as we camped there for days without leaving. We had entertainment and speeches, and we gathered daily to encourage each other to keep up the fight. We named ourselves "The Village," and another student leader and I published a daily newsletter to let the rest of the student body know exactly what we were fighting for. It was the closest thing to being alive during the seventies era that I felt. We ate together at various downtown businesses that donated food for us as soon as they realized what we were fighting for. Midway through the sit-in, the body of a young black man was found in a wooded area near Mount Nittany. The university tried to cover it up—they tried to play it off like it was not the body of a student and not connected to the threats in any way. Soon CNN showed up and interviewed students. It inserted a different type of energy into our building revolution. This stuff was real. It was serious. We were fighting for our lives. We were all over the news.

The student leader who had received the threats was wearing a bulletproof vest. We were informed that the FBI was on campus and conducting interviews. I was interviewed for *Rolling Stone* magazine about our campus climate.

One night when Raye and I were leaving the student union to grab something from home, a male student approached us and began screaming horrible things at us. I was terrified as he spewed hate all over us, calling us dykes and saying we were going to hell. We ran away from him and filed a police report about it, but he was never caught because we didn't know who he was, and on a campus of more than 40,000 students, it wasn't like we would have an opportunity to catch him. It was a scary time, and every time Raye and I would walk on campus we were emotionally guarded, our senses sharp to every sound around us. The thought that someone might actually harm us felt possible. I didn't let the fear get to me, and I was determined not only to not be affected by it, but to try to use it to create change on the campus and possibly in the world.

After the ten-day sit-in, university officials came around to meet our requests. The "Plan to Enhance Diversity at Penn State" established an African Studies Research Center in 2001–2002 and committed $900,000 in funding for the center over the following five-year period. The plan also required the university to have at least ten full-time faculty members in the African and African-American Studies department. We fought for the inclusion of an actual LGBT resource center, because at the time all we had was Dr. Rankin's tiny office. Two years later, they opened the doors to a beautiful center for lesbian, gay, bisexual, and transgender students. I was the first intern at the center. We made history at Penn State and proved that students do have power at a university. Protest worked, and a more diverse Penn State was the legacy that we created for the students who followed us.

I hadn't been to a meeting in the ten days that I had spent on campus, and that was the longest I had gone without a meeting in my entire recovery. I felt slightly out of touch and disjointed. I walked into a meeting after having gone through this major emotional upheaval, and everything everyone shared seemed so trivial compared to what I had just experienced. I went to open my mouth up to share, but I couldn't find the words to express myself. Where did I begin? How did I even begin to verbalize my feelings? For the first time in my recovery, I couldn't share my feelings in the meeting.

I went home that night feeling more confused than ever. I hadn't felt blocked in recovery before. I had always been able to explain my feelings; after all, it was recovery that enabled me to get in touch with them again. I knew I had to get this out of me—whatever it was—all the confusion, anger, frustration, and sadness that I felt over everything that had occurred. An idea began to form inside my head, one that would enable me to creatively express the emotions I felt during that time. And in a few moments, I began to write down what would become an art project called the Family Flag Project. It consisted of rainbow flags made up of individually colored panels that people would make, and then the panels would be sewn together to make up the flags. The exhibit depicted acts of violence and discrimination toward queer people, and I began traveling all across the East Coast to conferences and universities, doing workshops on hate crime and discrimination. The goal of the project was to give victims a method of healing using art—much like the AIDS Quilt or Clothesline Project—that would also serve as a visual awareness piece. I did this for more than two years and ended up with almost seven flags—over 250 individual panels created. It was my response to everything that had happened on campus. It was then that I realized I could utilize other tools to help me process my feelings in recovery. Maybe I couldn't always articulate what was happening to me and what I was feeling, but I still knew at a core level that I had to process it in order to stay healthy and maintain my recovery.

41

THREATS AND INSTANT MESSAGES

SUMMER CAME AND WENT, AND THE TENSIONS AND
acts of hate seemed to dissipate a little bit. Raye, who was majoring in
education to become a teacher, was required to do an internship at a
school for the entire semester. She was placed at a school about four
hours outside of Philadelphia. She came home every weekend, but it
was hard to have her away. Over the summer we had managed to get a
car with some money we had both saved from working. It was an older
model black Mazda, and it got us where we needed to be. I made sure I
surrounded myself with my college friends and went to meetings with
my brother as much as possible.

Things were quieting down on campus, but I still wasn't thrilled
being alone in our home, and I found myself once again sleeping with
the light on.

I spent the fall semester staying as busy as I could working on my internship in the center and going to more meetings than I had the previous semester. It was hard for me to walk into a meeting and listen to everyday issues when I felt that much heavier issues were occurring in my own life and on campus. Many of the student leaders I grew so close to had moved on and graduated, and it was becoming clear that I, too, would soon be moving on. I was excited and ready, but also unsure and sad. I had made such amazing strides in this small town; I had really grown up and built my recovery foundation here. My brother was now here, and the thought of staying did enter my mind, but I wasn't sure what I would be able to do for work.

The semester went by quickly, and before I knew it, Christmas break had come and Raye was home. Spring semester started with the realization that this would be my last semester as a college student. It was exciting and sad, and just when I thought things were quiet on campus—something happened that knocked the wind out of me.

In April of 2002, I came home from school one day to find the message light blinking on my answering machine. The message went something like this: "Hello, my name is Bill and I work for the Anti-Defamation League in Philadelphia. I came across some disturbing information about you today on a nationally known hate group's web page, and I am concerned for your safety. I need you to call me back right away." I just stared at the machine in shock. I was home alone and it was dark out, and I started to panic a bit. I called him back immediately, and he explained that it was his job to track online hate group activity for this organization and that he had come across a web page dedicated to me. My full name, my address, my home phone number, and the words "queen dyke at Penn State" were on the page. It went on to say that I was a sodomite who held gay pride rallies on campus and that I should be dealt with accordingly.

Apparently this particular hate group (that I will not name so as not to give any credence to their status in this world) was famously known for creating what was commonly referred to as the "lone wolf activity." This group, which was led by an attorney and knew the law well, would provide basic information about people they didn't like to anyone who came upon their web page and insinuate that someone should do something violent to these people. This group hated anyone who wasn't a white Christian. People would surf onto the web page to find the targets, and then, on their own accord, commit a hate crime against the people listed on the page. It was a clever way to initiate hate activity; the owner of the group was never able to be held accountable because all he did was provide what was considered public information about people and express his feelings toward them—which, of course, was his First Amendment right.

So here I sat, on the phone with a guy telling me all this information and saying that I would most likely start receiving hate mail or death threats. He told me to report anything I received immediately to the police and to call him back if I did in fact get anything. Sure enough, as I hung up the phone and sat down at my computer to check my e-mail, there was an e-mail that read, "Death to all queers, you shall die by my hand," from an AOL address I had never seen before. I immediately picked up the phone and called Raye who told me to call the police, which I did as she made her way home. I told the police what happened and they asked me to come downtown to file a report. I told them I would be down as soon as Raye arrived home. I was shaking as I waited for Raye. I went to the web site the guy told me about and saw the page about me and noticed that it also listed three of my friends. There was a chat room at the bottom of the page, and I saw the same AOL address that sent the death threat to me via e-mail. The person had a profile on the page that simply said, "On a perch with my rifle waiting." I instant-messaged my friend, who was also listed on the web site, and she also had received an e-mail. I called the other two friends, and they had the same message waiting for them. I told them to meet me at the police station.

I spent the next three hours at the police station with my friends as we all filed our complaints. The police said they would try to contact AOL and track the message. I thought it was pretty stupid for someone to send a death threat via AOL, but given the mentality of anyone who would expound such hate toward another, I guess it didn't surprise me. The police reported the incident to university officials, and I found myself on the phone with the vice provost, who said the university president was deeply concerned about this incident and would do whatever it took to get to the bottom of it. In the meantime, they would check in with me periodically and the campus police would do wellness checks by our house.

After we finished up at the police station, Raye and I went to a computer lab on campus because we both had work to do and neither of us wanted to go home just yet. We were freaked out that our home address was now listed on a web page for any hate monger to find. We sat down and logged onto the computers and, as AOL Instant Messenger popped up, as it always did when I logged on to the computer—I had an idea. I thought if this person was dumb enough to e-mail me using an AOL account, he or she probably also used Instant Messenger. I decided to place the person's screen name on my buddy list—since the e-mail was an AOL account, I knew the screen name would be the e-mail address. Sure enough, as soon as I added the screen name to my buddy list, the name showed up as actively online. I froze, but instead of letting my fear get the best of me, I got pissed off. I decided to send the person a message asking them why they had sent me the e-mail. I typed, "Hi, this is the girl you sent a death threat to earlier today and I am just wondering why" and I hit send. I sat there waiting, and as I noticed the person was typing back, I called Raye over. I told her to call the police station right away and let them know what I was doing. The person, who never identified him- or herself, began a rant that lasted over fifteen minutes, describing in vivid detail the method that would be used to kill me. I kept responding with what I thought were rational questions, like "You don't even know me, why would you want to hurt me?" The person went on about how all gays were sinners and deserved to die. Raye was relaying everything to the police, who were on the other line with AOL trying to pinpoint the location of the individual I was speaking to. They needed me to keep this person on the computer as long as I could, which was getting harder to do as my hands were shaking. The person told me they would beat me to a bloody pulp and tie me to a fence like Matthew Shepard for the world to watch me die. At this point I was crying, and I no longer had any words to respond. The person wrote, "I'm getting angry and I'm going to come and find you," and then signed off.

I just sat there, tears rolling down my face, my hands shaking and my head spinning. How could someone I don't even know want to hurt me in this way? Raye got off the phone and said that AOL had gotten a position on the person and the police would let us know what happened once they found him or her. We left the computer lab that night, and as we walked into our house, we were petrified. I flung on every light in the house. Every sound outside made me jump out of my skin. If I saw headlights shining through the window, my pulse quickened. I kept telling myself that it was okay and that we would be fine. Raye kept doing the same, but we both had a degree of fear and doubt in our voices and eyes that was impossible to mask. The next day, after not sleeping all night, we went on campus to speak to university officials. They informed us that they had contacted the person in charge of the web site and our information was taken down. They tracked the AOL conversation to a seventeen-year-old boy living in New Jersey who was in no way affiliated with Pennsylvania State University, which made the university officials ecstatic since it meant they avoided any potentially harmful press, even though the incident got plenty of press coverage across the state. I had reporters from Harrisburg and Pittsburgh calling me for information. I gave interviews because I wanted people to know what was going on and the hate that existed in the world. I wanted people to know me and know that I was a good person who didn't deserve this. Through all this, my recovery was tested. In my past, things like this were the driving forces behind my drinking and drugging, but not now. This event only made me stronger in my resolve. I wasn't going to be someone's victim. I wasn't going to relapse over this and lose everything I'd worked so hard for. That wasn't the person I was anymore. Instead, I decided to use the incident to fight back and create change. I couldn't believe a seventeen-year-old boy was behind all this, and it made my heart ache for him and his family. He was charged with seven counts for my incident alone, including being charged with a hate crime—a crime that I would come to find could not have been charged in the state of Pennsylvania, because our state's laws didn't include sexual orientation as a protected class. I used the Serenity Prayer in every aspect of my life and believed strongly in the part that says "the courage to change the things I can." This was something I could change, and I set out to do so.

42

A LIFE OF ACTIVISM

AFTER THE REALIZATION THAT THE HATE CRIME
charge couldn't have been added if the offender in my case had lived in
Pennsylvania, I decided I was going to do everything in my power to
help with the existing efforts to get a hate crime bill passed in the state.
I just couldn't fathom that this person's pure intent and motivation
for the crime against me was his hatred toward gay people. I began
working with my mentor, Dr. Rankin. She had helped form a statewide
coalition called the Statewide Pennsylvania Rights Coalition (SPARC)
that advocated for fully inclusive rights for all lesbian, bisexual, gay,
and transgender people. The coalition had no paid staff and was run by
representatives of other organizations throughout the state with similar
missions. They spoke in one unified voice to the legislature regarding
issues concerning gay rights. They had a student activism arm, and
I became the co-chair of the group. I learned a tremendous amount
about legislation, civil and legal rights, and victims' rights. SPARC

had been working for several years to push through an inclusive hate crime bill that would add sexual orientation, gender, gender identity, and mental and physical handicap to the existing bill. It would further add the wording "actual or perceived" before all the categories, because many crimes being committed in the state were based on one's perceived status.

I remember one time in State College when a fraternity brother was walking home after a party with a friend, and two guys approached them and started yelling insinuations that they were gay. The altercation led to an attack on one of the guys and left him with a fractured arm. He wasn't gay, but the offender thought he was, and that motivated the attack. Under the current law, the hate crime enhancement would not have been able to be included.

As graduation came into focus, it became abundantly clear by my passion and motivation that I was not going to become a drug and alcohol counselor. College and my experiences had molded me into an activist and advocate, and I wanted nothing more than to get a position to further my work in these areas. Raye and I graduated together, and my parents threw us a huge joint graduation party, which was one of the happiest days of my life. I got to wear a cap and gown for the first time ever and walk in a graduation ceremony, while my parents, brothers, and loving partner watched from afar. I was robbed of that experience in high school, having never been able to walk in graduation due to my delinquencies. It was an amazing feeling knowing that I broke a cycle in my family. I had broken the cycle of addiction, and I became the first person in my entire family to ever graduate from college. I felt so much pride in the moment when I walked on stage and accepted my degree. I felt so accomplished. I had finished something important in my life.

In the program they say that when the student is ready, the teacher will appear, and I believe my career teacher was Dr. Rankin. She informed me that SPARC had just received a grant that would enable them to hire their first full-time managing director, and she encouraged me to apply. I applied, interviewed, and was offered the job in Harrisburg, Pennsylvania. Only a few months after the drama and trauma of 9/11 and my own brush with hate crimes, Raye and I packed for our new life in Harrisburg. It felt like, once again, God's plan for me was being realized—I was being placed exactly where I was meant to be. It was also validating in a way to know that all the turmoil I went through on campus was for a reason. It was so I could move on and create more change in society.

It was sad for me to leave State College. I had undergone so much growth in that little town, had come so far, and had made such amazing friends who were my family. I knew that I would keep in touch with each and every one of them, but it would be different. I wouldn't be able to walk into a meeting and see them every week or walk into my college office and see my favorite boys and know that I had unconditional support all around me. I would have to rebuild that in Harrisburg. But I knew I would be okay, because throughout those years in State College, that was the one certainty recovery gave me. If I didn't pick up a drink or a drug on any given day—my life would be okay. And no matter what I was going through—I would be okay! That is the one great gift and promise of recovery.

Epilogue

IN 2002, SPARC DID HELP PASS THE MOST INCLUSIVE hate crimes legislation in the nation, and I was given an appointment by the governor, Edward G. Rendell, to serve as a commissioner for the Pennsylvania Commission on Crime and Delinquency. After the law's passage, I was given an opportunity to interview for an executive director position at a nonprofit agency that serves crime victims, and I got the job in 2003. I continue to serve as both a commissioner and the executive director of the Victim/Witness Assistance Program. I am living my life's purpose, and it is with great pride and joy that I do so.

My earlier premonitions about Raye were correct, and she and I did end up getting married; however, it was a short-lived union. We were young and both not quite ready for all that we tried to have. We still remain very close friends and share custody of our dog Tanner. Magi is still in my life and serves as my sponsor, mentor, best friend, and sister. We speak daily and continue to learn so much from each other. My second sponsor, Rose, was killed suddenly one day while pulling out of her driveway. It was a freak accident; a truck was traveling past her home and she did not see it as she backed out. I was devastated. She was a wonderful lady and provided so much of the foundation of my recovery. I miss her and think of her all the time.

I would have none of the experiences and accomplishments in life that I have today without recovery. I am one of the lucky ones; I got into recovery at a young age, and to this day have managed not to pick up a drink or a drug. I still go to meetings. I still call my sponsor. I still read recovery literature because recovery is a lifelong journey. I treasure and protect my recovery with the fierce knowledge that without it, I have and am nothing. You can do anything and get through anything without using. I am living proof of that. I try to spread the message of hope to many others I encounter that recovery is an option and it can create a life beyond your wildest expectations if you allow it to. It has for me, and it can for you. So keep doing the next right thing and enjoy the ride. I sure as hell am!

Resource Guide

These are just a few resources for you to seek out in case you need assistance as I did in early recovery.

Alcoholics Anonymous
www.aa.org

Gay, Lesbian and Straight Network
www.glsen.org

In the Rooms
www.intherooms.com

Narcotics Anonymous
www.na.org

National Organization of Victim Assistance
www.trynova.org

Rape Abuse Incest National Network
www.rainn.org

The Second Road
www.thesecondroad.org

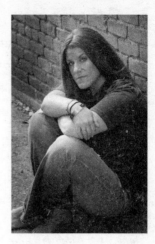

JENNIFER STORM, AUTHOR
LEAVE THE LIGHT ON

JENNIFER STORM WAS BORN AND RAISED NEAR Allentown, Pennsylvania and attended Northampton High School. She graduated from Pennsylvania State University with a Bachelor of Science in Rehabilitation Services and a Master's Degree in Organizational Management from The University of Phoenix.

In August 2002, Ms. Storm joined Victim-Witness Assistance Program (VWAP) as the organization's second Executive Director. Before joining VWAP, Ms. Storm was the first full-time director of the Statewide Pennsylvania Rights Coalition, a nonprofit coalition dedicated to securing and defending fully inclusive civil rights for LGBT people in Pennsylvania. During her tenure at Pennsylvania Rights Coalition, Ms. Storm worked diligently on obtaining inclusive hate crime legislation.

In 2002, the Pennsylvania legislature passed one of the most inclusive hate crime statutes in the country. Governor Edward G. Rendell appointed Ms. Storm as a commissioner to the Pennsylvania Commission on Crime and Delinquency. She was later appointed to the Homeland Security, Law Enforcement and Justice Systems Advisory committees where she also serves on the Terrorism Prevention and Local Law Enforcement Subcommittee.

Ms. Storm is active in many local committees and on boards such as: The Greater Harrisburg Foundation EGAL Board, Dauphin County Domestic Violence Taskforce, Joint Investigative Taskforce, Dauphin County Elder Abuse Taskforce, Northern Dauphin Human Services Advisory Panel, and Criminal Justice Advisory Board of Dauphin County.

Her media appearances are vast and include frequent appearances on all major networks, including ABC, FOX, NBC, NPR, CBS, and PBS as the county spokesperson for victims' rights. She has been featured in *Curve Magazine, The Advocate, Time Magazine, Rolling Stone, WE Magazine for Women, Women Magazine,* and many more.

Recently, Ms. Storm was selected to appear on the cover of *WE Magazine for Women.* The selection was based on her business acumen, community service, and life experiences, as well as her compelling story of triumph over tragedy. Her story was featured in the magazine's Fall 2009 issue.

This is Ms. Storm's second memoir. Her first memoir, *Blackout Girl: Growing Up and Drying Out in America,* was published in 2008 by Hazelden.